Infection Challenges in the Critical Care Unit

Editor

MAY MEI-SHENG RILEY

CRITICAL CARE NURSING CLINICS OF NORTH AMERICA

www.ccnursing.theclinics.com

Consulting Editor
CYNTHIA BAUTISTA

December 2021 • Volume 33 • Number 4

ELSEVIER

1600 John F. Kennedy Boulevard • Suite 1800 • Philadelphia, Pennsylvania, 19103-2899

http://www.theclinics.com

CRITICAL CARE NURSING CLINICS OF NORTH AMERICA Volume 33, Number 4
December 2021 ISSN 0899-5885, ISBN-13: 978-0-323-84910-4

Editor: Kerry Holland
Developmental Editor: Ann Gielou M. Posedio

Critical Care Nursing Clinics of North America (ISSN 0899-5885) is published quarterly by Elsevier Inc., 360 Park Avenue South, New York, NY 10010-1710. Months of issue are March, June, September, and December. Business and Editorial Offices: 1600 John F. Kennedy Blvd., Suite 1800, Philadelphia, PA 19103-2899. Periodicals postage paid at New York, NY and additional mailing offices. Subscription prices are $160.00 per year for US individuals, $576.00 per year for US institutions, $100.00 per year for US students and residents, $206.00 per year for Canadian individuals, $596.00 per year for Canadian institutions, $230.00 per year for international individuals, $596.00 per year for international institutions, $115.00 per year for international students/residents and $100.00 per year for Canadian students/residents. To receive student/resident rate, orders must be accompanied by name of affiliated institution, data of term, and the *signature* of program/residency coordinator on institution letterhead. Orders will be billed at individual rate until proof of status is received. Foreign air speed delivery is included in all *Clinics* subscription prices. All prices are subject to change without notice. **POSTMASTER:** Send address changes to *Critical Care Nursing Clinics of North America*, Elsevier Health Sciences Division, Subscription Customer Service, 3251 Riverport Lane, Maryland Heights, MO 63043. **Customer Service: 1-800-654-2452 (US and Canada); 314-447-8871 (outside US and Canada). Fax: 314-447-8029. E-mail:** JournalsCustomerService-usa@elsevier.com **(for print support) and** JournalsOnlineSupport-usa@elsevier.com **(for online support).**

Reprints. For copies of 100 or more of articles in this publication, please contact the Commercial Reprints Department, Elsevier Inc., 360 Park Avenue South, New York, New York, 10010-1710; Tel.: 212-633-3874, Fax: 212-633-3820, and E-mail: reprints@elsevier.com.

Critical Care Nursing Clinics of North America is covered in *MEDLINE/PubMed (Index Medicus), International Nursing Index, Nursing Citation Index, Cumulative Index to Nursing and Allied Health Literature,* and *RNdex Top 100.*

Contributors

CONSULTING EDITOR

CYNTHIA BAUTISTA, PhD, APRN, FNCS, FCNS
Associate Professor, Egan School of Nursing and Health Studies, Fairfield University, Fairfield, Connecticut, USA

EDITOR

MAY MEI-SHENG RILEY, MSN, MPH, RN, ACNP, CCRN, CIC, FAPIC
Area Director, Infection Prevention and Control, Department of Infection Prevention and Control, Providence Saint Joseph Health System, Northern California–Humboldt, Infection Control Consultant, Department of Infection Prevention and Control, Stanford Health Care, Stanford, California, USA

AUTHORS

MICHAEL H. ACKERMAN, DNS, RN, FCCM, FNAP, FAANP, FAAN
Director, Masters in Healthcare Innovation Program, Professor of Clinical Nursing, The Ohio State University, Columbus, Ohio, USA

THOMAS AHRENS, PhD, RN, FAAN
Founder, Viven Health, St Louis, Missouri, USA

IRIS BERMAN, MSN, BSN, RN, CCRN-K
VP, Telehealth Services, Northwell Health, Syosset, New York, USA

TOM BOBICH, MBA
VP - Marketing, Hicuity Health, Irvine, California, USA

THERESA BRINDISE, MS, BSN, RN
AdvocateAuroraHealth, Director, eICU, Oak Brook, Illinois, USA

CATHY C. CARTWRIGHT, DNP, RN-BC, PCNS, FAAN
Children's Mercy Kansas City, Kansas City, Missouri, USA

JIYEON CHOI, PhD, RN
Assistant Professor, Yonsei University College of Nursing, Mo-Im Kim Nursing Research Institute, Seoul, Korea

THERESA DAVIS, PhD, RN, NE-BC, FAAN
Clinical Operations Director, enVision TeleICU Inova Telemedicine, Inova Transfer Center, Falls Church, Virginia, USA

ANNEMARIE FLOOD, RN, BSN, MPH, CIC, FAPIC
Executive Director, Quality, Infection Prevention and Employee Health, City of Hope National Medical Center, Duarte, California, USA

ARIEL GILBERT, BSN, RN, CCRN
Children's Mercy Kansas City, Kansas City, Missouri, USA

LORA JENKINS-LONIDIER, DNP, ACNP-BC, FNP-BC, CCRN
Acute Care Nurse Practitioner, Administrative NP, Jackson Pulmonary Associates, Jackson, Jackson, Mississippi, USA

JUSTIN KELLY, MHI, BSN, RN, CCRN, RHIA
Staff Nurse, James Medical Intensive Care Unit, Ohio State University Comprehensive Cancer Center–Arthur G. James Cancer Hospital and Richard J. Solove Research Institute, Columbus, Ohio, USA

MAY MEI-SHENG RILEY, MSN, MPH, RN, ACNP, CCRN, CIC, FAPIC
Area Director, Infection Prevention and Control, Department of Infection Prevention and Control, Providence Saint Joseph Health System, Northern California–Humboldt, Infection Control Consultant, Department of Infection Prevention and Control, Stanford Health Care, Stanford, California, USA

RITA OLANS, DNP, RN, CPNP, APRN-BC, FNAP
Assistant Professor, School of Nursing, MGH Institute of Health Professions, Boston, Massachusetts, USA

ANNE PONTILLO, MHI, BSN, RN, CCRN
Staff Development Coordinator, James Critical Care, Ohio State University Comprehensive Cancer Center–Arthur G. James Cancer Hospital and Richard J. Solove Research Institute, Columbus, Ohio, USA

TERESA RINCON, PhD, RN, CCRN-K, FCCM
Assistant Professor, Graduate School of Nursing, University of Massachusetts Medical School, Worcester, MA, USA

JUDITH A. TATE, PhD, RN
Assistant Professor, Center of Healthy Aging, Self-Management and Complex Care, Director, Undergraduate Nursing Honors Program, The Ohio State University College of Nursing, Columbus, Ohio, USA

CINDY WELSH, RN, MBA, FACHE
VP, Adult Critical Care, eICU, Advocate Intensivist Partners, AdvocateAuroraHealth, Oak Brook, Illinois, USA

Contents

The continuing rise in the incidence of multidrug-resistant organism infections has made combating this grave threat a national imperative. One of the most potent weapons in our arsenal against such organisms is the prudent use of antibiotics. Antimicrobial stewardship (AMS) programs aim to slow the development of antimicrobial resistance through judicious, monitored use of antibiotics. Traditionally, AMS programs have included pharmacists and physicians with training in AWS, infectious disease physicians, hospital leadership, microbiologists, and infection prevention professionals. Nurses are missing from AMS programs, especially intensive care nurses. Critical care nurses provide the majority of patient care to ICU patients and monitor the progress of the patient's condition. The ICU nurse is an obvious asset to the AMS programs. ICU nurses are well-educated autonomous professionals with a unique role in coordinating with the critical care team. Critical care nurses already perform numerous nursing tasks with AWS functions. This, together with their unique perspective makes them a valuable asset that has often been overlooked. Traditionally, perceived barriers have kept ICU nurses from joining AMS teams. By removing these barriers and engaging critical care nurses in the important work of AWS, we can strengthen our AMS team and achieve optimal outcomes for our patients.

Pneumonia is a leading cause of morbidity and mortality and a primary cause of hospitalizations. Guidelines have been established through the American Thoracic Society and Infectious Diseases Society of America in 2016 focusing on the causative pathogen for antibiotic selection. In 2017 an International European task force provided guidelines of specific antibiotic selections based on drug resistance and mortality risk. Improving patient outcomes is based not only on the appropriate treatment, which should not be delayed, but also on implementation and adherence to evidence-based strategies to reduce the increased risk of mortality.

Most fungal infections are common in humans. Pathogenic fungi are opportunistic but can cause fungal infection disease in patients with immunocompromised conditions, such as malignancy, chemotherapy, transplantation, acquired immunodeficiency syndrome, and usage of immunosuppressant drugs. Most invasive infections are caused by Aspergillus species, mucormycetes, Cryptococcus species, and Candida species. This article focuses on environmental fungi such as Aspergillus species and mucormycetes because the mode of transmission is different. The purpose of this article is to discuss invasive fungal infections (IFIs) caused by environmental fungi and to educate critical care nurses about infection control and risk mitigation to prevent IFIs.

This article provides an overview of the history of the sepsis definitions as well as an overview of the current understanding of the pathogenesis of sepsis. The evolution of the treatment bundles is also presented.

Currently, the Centers for Disease Control reports close to 40,000 central line–associated bloodstream infections (CLABSI) occur in acute care facilities in the United States each year. Most are considered preventable. Evidence-based practices such as the CLABSI bundle and central line maintenance bundles have demonstrated their effectiveness in reducing CLABSI. This article reviews these best practices and provides a framework for consistent implementation.

Hospital-acquired central line–associated bloodstream infections (CLABSIs) are the leading cause of infections in the pediatric intensive care unit. Bacteria responsible for CLABSIs are spread by health care workers, parents, and families and mitigated by scrupulous attention to hand hygiene and safety prevention strategies. Maintenance bundles are grouped elements, such as hand hygiene, standardized dressing and tubing changes, and aseptic technique for entering a central line, effective in preventing CLABSIs. Nurses can decrease the incidence of CLABSIs by using maintenance bundles and including parents and families in safety prevention strategies.

Special Articles

JiYeon Choi and Judith A. Tate

> Communication is a critical component of patient-centered care. Critically ill, mechanically ventilated patients are unable to speak and this condition is frightening, frustrating, and stressful. Impaired communication in the intensive care unit (ICU) contributes to poor symptom identification and restricts effective patient engagement. Older adults are at higher risk for communication impairments in the ICU because of pre-illness communication disorders and cognitive dysfunction that often accompanies or precedes critical illness. Assessing communication disorders and developing patient-centered strategies to enhance communication can lessen communication difficulty and increase patient satisfaction.

Cindy Welsh, Teresa Rincon, Iris Berman, Tom Bobich, Theresa Brindise, and Theresa Davis

> Telehealth in intensive care units (TeleICU) is the provision of critical care using audio-visual communication and health information systems across varying clinical and geographically dispersed settings. The optimal structure of a TeleICU team is one that leverages expert clinical knowledge to address the needs of critical care patients, regardless of hospital location or availability of an onsite intensivist. Information related to the optimal TeleICU team structure is lacking. This article examines the optimal TeleICU team composition, which is one that incorporates the use of an interdisciplinary approach, leverages technology, and is cognizant of varying geographic locations.

CRITICAL CARE NURSING
CLINICS OF NORTH AMERICA

SERIES OF RELATED INTEREST

Nursing Clinics of North America http://www.nursing.theclinics.com
Advances in Family Practice Nursing www.advancesinfamilypracticenursing.com

---

THE CLINICS ARE AVAILABLE ONLINE!
Access your subscription at:
www.theclinics.com

Preface

Infection Control and Prevention Considerations for the Intensive Care Unit

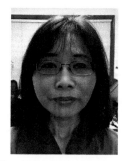

May Mei-Sheng Riley, MSN, MPH, RN, ACNP, CCRN, CIC, FAPIC
Editor

Intensive care unit (ICU)-associated infections are those that occur 48 hours after ICU admission. These can lead to significant morbidity and mortality. Of these, blood-stream and pulmonary infections have the highest mortality.

Critical care patients are more likely to have extended ICU stays and prolonged hospitalization. ICU-associated infections significantly impact quality of care and patient safety. The consequences of Hospital-associated infections (HAIs), including economic burdens and social expenses, are overwhelming to patients, their families, and health care facilities.

Modern critical care units house a unique mixture of the most severely ill patients with multiple comorbidities having various invasive medical catheters and tubing, taking immunosuppressant drugs, and requiring advanced medical technologies to save their lives. Infections acquired in the ICU setting have become common, occurring in nearly one in 10 critically ill hospitalized patients.

It is imperative that critical care nurses recognize the detrimental impact of HAIs. Aggressive infection control measures must be implemented and enforced to limit the incidence of ICU-associated infections. Researchers, public health authorities, and professional organization committees have developed and continue to create evidence-based practice guidelines to eliminate ICU infections. A multifaceted approach is essential and should include infection prevention committees, antimicrobial stewardship programs, daily assessments of infection prevention practice bundles, identification and minimization of modifiable risk factors, efforts to increase awareness, and continuing nursing education programs. Infection control in the critical care setting is

Crit Care Nurs Clin N Am 33 (2021) ix–x
https://doi.org/10.1016/j.cnc.2021.09.003
0899-5885/21/© 2021 Published by Elsevier Inc.

ccnursing.theclinics.com

an evolving field of research for patient safety and quality of care in the critical care patient population.

Necessary for success in preventing ICU infections is dedicated leadership, including a hospital epidemiologist with background in infectious disease, a microbiologist, an infection prevention nurse, pharmacists, critical care nurses, and information technicians. Critical care nurses are often key partners in infection prevention, as HAIs tend to focus on critical care settings. The infection prevention program has several functions, such as surveillance, surveillance data management, education for critical care clinicians, isolation implementation, hand hygiene compliance promotion, and evaluation of its compliance, along with developing infection prevention protocols for bundle practice. Effectiveness is assessed by continued use of data to drive and sustain performance, monitoring of outcomes and performance evaluation of infection prevention procedures.

May Mei-Sheng Riley, MSN, MPH, RN, ACNP, CCRN, CIC, FAPIC
Department of Infection Prevention and Control
Providence Saint Joseph Health System
Northern California–Humboldt
Department of Infection Prevention and Control
Stanford Health Care
300 Pasteur Drive
Room H0105, M/C 5221
Stanford, CA 94305-5623, USA

E-mail address:
mriley@stanfordhealthcare.org

Implementing an Antimicrobial Stewardship Program in the Intensive Care Unit by Engaging Critical Care Nurses

May Mei-Sheng Riley, MSN, MPH, RN, ACNP, CCRN, CIC, FAPIC[a,b],*,
Rita Olans, DNP, RN, CPNP, APRN-BC, FNAP[c]

KEYWORDS

- Antimicrobial stewardship • Multidrug-resistant organisms (MDRO) • Critical care
- Engagement

KEY POINTS

- MDROs are a serious public health threat.
- Antimicrobial stewardship is an evidence-based strategy to combat this threat.
- Currently, antimicrobial stewardship programs do not include nurses.
- Critical care nurses provide the majority of patient care to ICU patients and monitor the progress of the patient's condition. They would be a valuable asset to the ASP team.
- Critical care nurses should be included in ASPs to achieve optimal patient outcomes.

INTRODUCTION

Since the discovery of penicillin, excessive and indiscriminate use of antimicrobial agents has led to the selection of organisms with resistance to many antibiotics. Multidrug-resistant organisms (MDROs) limit antimicrobial treatment options and, in some cases, have no option for treatment.

The Centers for Disease Control and Prevention (CDC) estimates that drug-resistant bacteria cause 23,000 deaths and 2 million infections annually in the United States.[1] Burnham and colleagues[2] report that these numbers likely underestimate the actual numbers, estimating the true number of deaths to be between 153,113 and 162,044. This places infections resistant to treatment as the third leading cause of death in the United States for the year 2010.[3] The CDC has identified antimicrobial resistance as one of the most important public health threats in the United States.[4]

Funding and financial disclosure: Nothing to disclose.
[a] Providence Saint Joseph Health System, 2700 Dolbeer Street, Eureka, CA 95501, USA;
[b] Stanford Health Care, 300 Pasteur Drive, Room H0105, M/C 5221, Stanford, CA 94305-5623, USA; [c] MGH Institute of Health Professions, School of Nursing, 36 First Avenue, Boston, MA 02128, USA
* Corresponding author.
E-mail addresses: mriley@stanfordhealthcare.org; mayriley@gmail.com

Crit Care Nurs Clin N Am 33 (2021) 369–380
https://doi.org/10.1016/j.cnc.2021.07.001
0899-5885/21/© 2021 Elsevier Inc. All rights reserved.

Rapid MDRO emergence and dissemination in critical care settings has become a serious health issue worldwide.[5] The causes of antimicrobial resistance development are multifactorial. Selective pressure resulting from antimicrobial agent exposure and inappropriate antimicrobial usage directly contributes to the growing challenge of MDRO development in critical care settings.[5,6] Antimicrobial stewardship (AMS) programs are currently the best available approach to antibiotic use in the setting of such drug resistance. Several articles already discuss the important AMS roles played by nurses and the importance of their inclusion in AMS teams.[7–12] The central role of intensive care unit (ICU) nurse-driven interventions include numerous functions integral to the successful operation of AMS programs.[13,14]

The purpose of this article is to (1) discuss the need for critical care nurses to engage in AMS initiatives and strategies to combat antibiotic resistance, (2) delineate the AMS activities that ICU nurses already perform, and (3) discuss supportive strategies that can assist ICU nurses in becoming key members of AMS efforts.

The terms "antibiotic stewardship" and "antimicrobial stewardship" are different, although they have been frequently used interchangeably. Antibiotics are regimens that specifically target bacteria. However, microbes include not just bacteria, but also viruses, fungi, and parasites. Antimicrobials refer to agents that treat all these pathogens. The term "antimicrobial stewardship" will be used throughout the article and includes the larger scope of pathogens that can infect ICU patients.

The Necessity of Antimicrobial Stewardship Programs in Intensive Care Units

In 2013, the CDC published a comprehensive analysis, entitled Antibiotic Resistance Threats in the United States, delineating the top 18 antibiotic-resistant organisms in the United States.[15] Conscientious antibiotic stewardship is essential to combat these emergent threats and to avert a return to a preantibiotic era without effective chemotherapy. Infection control strategies are directed at the prevention of transmission of MDROs among patients while AMS focuses broadly on limiting the overuse of antimicrobial agents that can enhance the emergence of drug-resistant organisms.

The rate of multiresistant hospital-associated infections (HAIs) occurring in ICUs is higher than in noncritical care units in part because ICU patients are more likely to be exposed to antimicrobial regimens in critical care settings. According to a multistate HAI prevalence study, 9.1% of patients develop HAIs while receiving care in ICUs compared to a 3.1% HAI rate in admissions to all other units.[16] Analysis of pediatric data from the European Centre for Disease Prevention and Control demonstrates that pediatric ICUs (15.5%, 95% confidence interval, 11.6–20.3) and neonatal ICUs (10.7%, 9.0–12.7) have higher prevalence rates of HAI compared with pediatric surgery wards (3.4%, 2.3–4.9), neonatology wards (3.5%, 2.8–4.5), and general pediatric wards (1.8%, 1.4–2.4).[17]

Given the severity of illness in patients in ICUs, careful thought must be given to how to judiciously use antimicrobials in the critical care setting. Appropriate antibiotic stewardship includes optimal treatment of infections (ie, right drug, right time, right dose, right duration of therapy)[18] and improvement of antimicrobial prescription to (1) avoid ordering unnecessary broad-spectrum antibiotics, (2) shorten the treatment duration, (3) reduce undue antimicrobial usage, and (4) prevent adverse outcomes such as antimicrobial resistance, drug toxicity, and Clostridioides difficile (C difficile). infection.[18,19] Such AMS interventions have been shown to achieve equivalent patient outcomes without increased morbidity or mortality.[20]

Research studies reveal that 30% to 60% of antibiotic prescriptions in ICUs are unnecessary, inappropriate, or suboptimally dosed.[5] A prospective, multinational pharmacokinetic point-prevalence study involving 361 ICU patients examined the correlation between the unbound plasma concentrations of β-lactam antibiotics and patient outcome across 68 hospitals.[21] This study discovered that of the 248 ICU patients treated with β-lactam antibiotics for infection, 16% of the patients did not achieve minimum conservative pharmacokinetic/pharmacodynamic targets and these patients were 32% less likely to have a positive clinical outcome.[21]

Antimicrobial Stewardship and Intensive Care Unit Nurses

The goals of an AMS program are to (1) promote judicious use of antimicrobials by selecting the appropriate regimen, dose, duration, and route of administration; (2) stop or slow the development of organism drug resistance; (3) maximize the therapeutic outcome; and (4) minimize side effects and adverse drug reactions.[22] Originally, a typical AMS team has included pharmacists and physicians with training in AMS, infectious disease physicians, microbiologists, and infection prevention professionals supported by administration.[23] Unfortunately, registered nurses have often been overlooked. However, many studies have posited that nurse inclusion in AMS could help improve clinical outcomes as many nursing tasks and patient care activities already align with AMS interventions.[7,24]

In 2014, the CDC published its Core Elements of Hospital Antibiotic Stewardship Programs.[25] This includes 7 components: leadership commitment, accountability, drug expertise, action, tracking, reporting, and education. These key principles are designed to improve patient outcomes by guiding health care providers in judicious, appropriate use of antimicrobials. **Table 1**.

Recently, professional organizations including the CDC, American Nurses Association (ANA), Association for Professionals in Infection Control and Epidemiology (APIC), Society for Healthcare Epidemiology of America (SHEA), and Infectious Diseases Society of America (IDSA) have acknowledged the need for health care facilities to commit to forming antibiotic stewardship programs that incorporate the CDC's core elements.[25,26] In March 2015, the Obama Administration released the National Action

Table 1
Seven components in the CDC's Core Elements of Hospital Antibiotic Stewardship Programs

Summary of Core Elements of Hospital Antibiotic Stewardship Programs[25]	
Leadership Commitment	Dedicating Necessary Human, Financial and Information Technology Resources.
Accountability	Appointing a single leader responsible for program outcomes. Experience with successful programs shows that a physician leader is effective.
Drug Expertise	Appointing a single pharmacist leader responsible for working to improve antibiotic use.
Action	Implementing at least one recommended action, such as systemic evaluation of ongoing treatment needed after a set period of initial treatment (ie, "antibiotic time-outs" after 48 h).
Tracking	Monitoring antibiotic prescription and resistance patterns.
Reporting	Regular reporting of information on antibiotic use and resistance to doctors, nurses, and relevant staff.
Education	Educating clinicians about resistance and optimal prescription.

Data from Core Elements of Hospital Antibiotic Stewardship Programs. Atlanta, GA: US Department of Health and Human Services, CDC; 2014. Centers for Disease Control and Prevention Web site. http://www.cdc.gov/getsmart/healthcare/implementation/core-elements.html. Last updated February 6, 2020. Accessed March 7, 2020. https://www.cdc.gov/antibiotic-use/core-elements/hospital.html March 19, 2021.

Plan for Combating Antibiotic-Resistant Bacteria.[27] In May 2016, National Quality Forum (NQF) published the Antibiotic Stewardship Playbook.[22] The rationale of engaging nurses in the performance of AMS activities in their daily nursing tasks is supported in these documents. In addition, the Joint Commission's (TJC) Antimicrobial Stewardship Standard expects nurses and nurse practitioners to participate in AMS programs.[28]

Regulators and accrediting agencies along with legislative bodies have already made AMS a greater priority in health care facilities. The Joint Commission (TJC) has adopted antibiotic stewardship policies. These Joint Commission Antimicrobial Stewardship Standards under Medication Management (MM. 09.01.01) became effective on January 1, 2017.[28] All health care providers are required to comply with the TJC National Patient Safety Goals (NPSG).[29] to reduce HAIs.[29] The TJC improvement project named "Reducing Clostridium difficile Infections" is an initiative to reduce the risk of healthcare-associated C difficile through early identification, antibiotic stewardship, and effective environmental hygiene practices.[30] National Patient Safety Goal No. 3 (03.06.01) is to improve the safety of medication use.[29] AMS incorporates evidence-based strategies to limit the development of drug resistance and to improve patient safety with antibiotic treatment. AMS can fulfill the TJC's goal to reduce C difficile and NPSG No. 3 (03.06.01).[29,30] As nurses are educated to promote such patient safety, they are natural participants in AMS programs.

Critical care nurses provide direct patient care to ICU patients and monitor patients' progress while they are being treated for infections. They observe firsthand the progress of a patient's clinical condition and collaborate with the other health care professionals in the patient's treatment. Critical care nurses participate in the daily ICU rounds. Furthermore, they compose the largest group among all critical care professionals and, importantly, have been performing many daily nursing activities that correlate with AMS functions. **Table 2.**[25] Such nursing functions have been unrecognized as contributions to antibiotic stewardship, even by the nurses themselves.[7,31]

Success Factor: Engaging Intensive Care Unit Nurses to Participate in Combating Antibiotics Resistance

To optimize the chance of success, AMS programs must include critical care nurses as they work most closely with the patients, providing hands-on care.[9] Several articles already discuss the important AMS roles played by nurses and the importance of their inclusion in AMS teams.[7-12,32]

Some of the most notable examples of stewardship successes operationalized by critical care nurses involve the reduction in central-line–associated blood-stream infections (CLABSIs)[13] and the reduction of MDROs in ICUs following CHG bathing.[33] Besides the daily nursing tasks with stewardship functions, critical care nurses engage in evidence-based bundle practices to prevent CLABSI,[34] catheter-associated urinary tract infection (CAUTI),[35] and C difficile.[36] Critical care nurses can perform Methicillin-Resistant Staphylococcus Aureus (MRSA) nasal screening to help guide appropriate antibiotic management of pneumonia in the ICU and to initiate isolation precautions as needed.[37] Their attention to infection prevention guidelines helps improve patient safety both by helping prevent HAIs and the need to use more and broader antibiotics.

In 2017, ANA/CDC copublished a White Paper encouraging such interprofessional collaboration.[32] The ANA/CDC White Paper delineates the roles that nurses already play in fulfilling antibiotic stewardship activities while performing their daily nursing functions. Other publications have also evaluated and characterized the benefits of interprofessional teamwork in the ICU setting.[38,39] Although some publications discuss the widespread overlap between routine nursing activities with stewardship

Table 2
Daily nursing activities with antimicrobial stewardship functions

Daily Nursing Activity	Antimicrobial Stewardship Function
Nurses take patient's history of adverse drug reaction and drug allergy.	Accurate antibiotic allergy history guides optimal antibiotic selection.
Nurses obtain medication history and current medication information.	Accurate drug usage history.
Nurses perform medication reconciliation and document this in the medical record.	Accurate medication information.
Nurses collect microbiology laboratory culture specimens using aseptic technique before starting antibiotics.	Obtain culture specimens appropriately to prevent specimen contamination. A microbiology laboratory report from high-quality specimen can guide antibiotic selection. Obtaining the specimen before administering antibiotics prevents false-negative results.
Nurses promptly notify treating providers of the culture results and sensitivity. Nurses update patient's results for renal function, liver function, and drug level to treating providers.	Antibiotic adjustment based on the microbiology laboratory results reduces the use of broad-spectrum therapy. De-escalation leads to improved antibiotic dosing, reduced antibiotic resistance, more appropriate antibiotic selection, and reduced adverse events.
Nurses receive antibiotic orders. Nurses verify the regimen/dose/time/route and drug allergy history. Nurses administer antibiotics in a timely manner.	Timely administration of appropriate antibiotics.
Nurses monitor any adverse drug events including diarrhea.	Antibiotic adjustment to reduce drug adverse and side effects.
Nurses detect early signs of infection (eg, sepsis) by promptly starting antibiotics.	Early identification of infection and early treatment.
The nurse is the primary person communicating with the other professionals and coordinating patient care at a transition of care.	Avoids unnecessary antibiotic orders.
Nurses monitor patients' capacity to take medicines orally.	Assists in deciding when to convert antibiotic from intravenous to oral therapy.
Nurses continue to educate patients and families for drug safety and side effects observation.	Patient education.
Nurses participate in "antibiotic time-outs."	Reassess antibiotic therapy after 2–3 d when the reports of microbiology culture and sensitivity become available. Review antibiotics any time the patient develops a new condition (eg, C difficile).

Data from Refs.[7,8,32]

functions,[7,24,38] other recent papers have begun to document the specific benefits of nurse involvement in the enhancement of ICU and telemetry unit patient care.[14,40,41] Qualitative research was conducted to explore the role of the ICU nurse in AMS programs.[14] In 2016, Huang allowed that measurement of CAUTI reduction in the ICU is difficult to measure because of confounding variables, but 2020 Dahlin's[42] research and intervention documented a significant decrease in catheter-associated UTIs in the acute care setting using nurse-driven protocols.[35] These findings have implications for practice, which, if recognized and supported by all health care stakeholders from ICU to hospital management, could improve AMS in this acute care area.[14] Four categories emerged from the analysis: organizational, advocacy, clinical, and collaborative roles.[14]

To attain greater success, AMS programs need innovative, multidisciplinary approaches including the involvement of frontline bedside nurses. Ha and colleagues[40] published a study in 2019 demonstrating significant reductions in antimicrobial and acid suppressant medication, and urinary catheter utilization after engaging nurses through bedside nurse-driven AMS and infection prevention rounds. In the 12-month intervention period, the nurse-driven rounds team reviewed a total of 472 cases on antimicrobial therapy, 480 cases on acid suppressants, 321 cases with a urinary catheter, and 61 cases with a central venous catheter over a total of 867 patients. Compared with the preintervention period, significant reductions in unit antimicrobial use (791.2 vs 697.1 days of therapy per 1000 patient-days; $P = .03$), acid suppressant use (708.1 vs 372.4 days of therapy per 1000 patient-days; $P = .0001$), urinary catheter use (0.3 vs 0.2 catheter-days per patient-day; $P = .002$), and central venous catheter use (0.2 vs 0.1 catheter-days per patient-day; $P = .06$) were observed.[40] His later study also demonstrates the utility of time-outs that integrate nursing AMS into daily ICU rounds.[41]

Current Intensive Care Unit Nursing Activities with Antimicrobial Stewardship Functions

Intensive care nurses are involved in all sectors of patient care including direct care and communication between all stakeholders. Numerous ICU nurses' daily tasks overlap with AMS functions that are integral to successful antibiotic stewardship.[7]

Nurses are skilled in interdisciplinary and interpersonal communication, especially in the ICU. This central role places nurses in a unique and important position in optimizing communication between all other AMS stakeholders.[43] (**Fig. 1**)

The variety of nursing activities with AMS implications are summarized in **Table 2**.[7,8,32,43] The following interventions are often initiated by bedside nurses[25]:

- Optimization of microbiology cultures: Recognizing indications for when cultures should be obtained and knowing and implementing proper techniques for reducing contamination when collecting cultures.
- Reviews of antimicrobial therapy with "timeouts" on daily rounds (a strategy to prompt clinicians to re-evaluate antibiotic appropriateness including the need for de-escalation and discontinuation)
- Nurses closely follow patient treatments and know how long a patient has been receiving antimicrobial therapy and are often the first providers to be notified of patients' laboratory results. Nurses play an important role in reporting the early and ongoing patient response to initial antimicrobial therapy regimens.
- Transitions from intravenous to oral administration of medication: Evaluating patients' ability to tolerate oral medication and making recommendations to switch to oral antimicrobials.

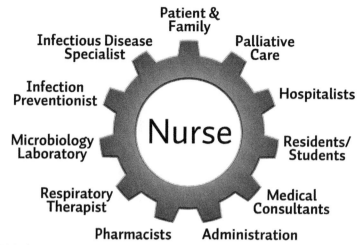

Fig. 1. Critical care Nurse communication related to antimicrobial stewardship. (*Data from* ANA & CDC. (2017). Redefining the Antibiotic Stewardship Team: Recommendations from the American Nurses Association/Centers for Disease Control and Prevention Workgroup on the Role of Registered Nurses in Hospital Antibiotic Stewardship Practices. Web site. https://www.cdc.gov/antibiotic-use/healthcare/pdfs/ANA-CDC-whitepaper.pdf   Published 2017. Accessed March 7, 2020. Last updated: July 2016. Accessed March 7, 2020 and Olans RD, Hausman NB, Olans RN. Nurses and antimicrobial stewardship: Past, present and future. Infect Dis Clin North Am. 2020; Mar;34(1):67-82.)

These contributions by critical care nurses to AMS have not yet been widely incorporated into all ASPs. However, there is growing recognition that bedside nurses have a vital role to play in AMS efforts.[7,10,25,32] These include the role of the nurse in diagnostic stewardship (eg, deciding if a patient's symptoms warrant obtaining a urine culture), verifying cultures are correctly performed before initiating antimicrobial treatment, improving specific penicillin allergy documentation, and initiating discussion of various aspects of antimicrobial treatment.[25]

Nurses already actively participate in many tasks with AMS functions (see **Table 2**).[7,8,32] These roles of ICU nurses in AMS programs have not yet been routinely incorporated in AMS programs. However, the recognition of daily ICU nursing activities with stewardship functions is evolving the roles that critical care nurses can play in stewardship.

Barriers and Gaps

Barriers to nurse AMS engagement have been identified and can be condensed as follows[7,8,24,32]:

- Nurses are not confident in reviewing microbiology laboratory results to determine antibiotic appropriateness since they lack microbiology training.[32]
- Nurses may not be familiar with antibiotic interactions, pharmacokinetics, and infusion rates of high-risk antibiotics, thus potentially posing a risk for adverse reactions.[44]
- Nurses are not familiar with the concepts and practice of AMS.[7,24,31,32]
- Nurses may not be aware of stewardship interventions and do not recognize that various nursing tasks have AMS benefits.[31]
- Hospital culture constrains nurses' AMS roles or excludes nurses from AMS participation.[24]

Table 3 Recommended action	
Antimicrobial Stewardship Barriers and Gaps	Strategic Action Plan
Lack of antimicrobial stewardship training Lack of confidence	Hospitals provide a didactic educational program for antimicrobial stewardship training.
Microbiologic knowledge gaps	Hospitals provide microbiology education: • How to interpret the laboratory culture results and sensitivity testing. • How to distinguish between infection and colonization.
Lack of stewardship perception	Hospitals illustrate the daily nursing activities with stewardship functions. • Stewardship means: conducting, supervising, or carefully managing of something entrusted to one's care. • Nurses are not antibiotic prescribers but are antibiotic stewards.
Lack of clearly defined nurses' stewardship roles	ASP leadership can define nurses' roles based on the daily nursing activities with stewardship functions.
Nurse exclusion Lack of culture for engaging nurses in ASPs	• Hospitals revise their antimicrobial stewardship policies to authorize the nurse roles in stewardship functions and include nurse representatives in the ASP committee and rounds. • Hospital leadership creates a culture of engaging nurses in stewardship. • Antimicrobial stewardship leadership includes nurse representatives in the antimicrobial stewardship meetings and rounds. • Hospitals empower antimicrobial stewardship champions at the patient care unit level.

Data from Refs.[8,24,25,31,32,40,45]

Nurses' lack confidence in their antibiotic and microbiological knowledge and have discomfort in discussing these issues with physicians.[24] These can be addressed through education and facility- and national-level hospital AMS policy revisions that delineate nursing functions and tasks related to antibiotic stewardship. Education[42] and culture change[24] can increase nurses' confidence and authority, thereby promoting nurses' engagement. Health care facility leadership must cultivate an environment that integrates nurses into ASPs and includes nursing representatives on AMS rounds.[45] A strategic action plan that focuses on removing the barriers is necessary to transition nurses to become critical members of the stewardship team.[32] These key recommendations for an action plan are summarized in **Table 3**.[8,24–26,31,32,45,46]

SUMMARY

MDRO infections in ICU patients lead to high morbidity and mortality, prolonged hospitalization, and increased medical expenses. There are also tangible human costs and emotional suffering. Combating antimicrobial-resistant organisms is a recognized national imperative.[27] AMS is a quality paradigm whose desired goal is optimal use of antimicrobials to accomplish a lower rate of drug resistance while achieving the best clinical outcomes. Experts in critical care have identified the critical importance of including effective AMS into the ICU setting.[20]

To succeed, actions to correct this multifaceted multidrug resistance problem must be comprehensive, accountable, sustained, and involve all sectors of the health care community. Many questions remain unanswered regarding the optimal management of antibiotic therapy for ICU patients.[47] For ASPs to achieve the best results, nursing professionals must be included in this effort. To sustain AMS in the ICU setting, Jeffs and colleagues[38] identify "leveraging the interest and passion of nurses, making it a routine practice, and engaging nurses to sustain and spread AMS practice by nurse leadership" as 3 key drivers of successful AS in the ICU setting.

Critical care nurses are well-trained and well-educated professionals who already perform a wide variety of AMS functions. They can be valuable contributors to these comprehensive AMS efforts. The success of multidisciplinary AMS will require an integrated, well-educated, interprofessional approach to the problem of antibiotic resistance.[48] In the most recent Society of Hospital Epidemiology of America White Paper on research needs in AMS, the authors acknowledge the need to evaluate the involvement of nurses in AMS activities in all health care settings.[49] Padigos and colleagues[50] have recently performed an elegant, detailed review of those studies describing nursing involvement in stewardship in the intensive care setting. More research will be necessary to identify and quantify the benefits of such nurse inclusion. Only by recognizing and better understanding each other's roles and contributions to AMS, we can create safer, more collaborative, and better integrated stewardship. In doing this, we can potentially decrease antimicrobial resistance in the ICU and improve critical care patient outcomes.[7]

CLINICS CARE POINTS

- Multidrug-resistant organisms (MDROs) are a serious public health issue worldwide.

- MDRO infection can increase mortality and morbidity and limit antimicrobial treatment options. It is imperative that we stop or slow the development of organism drug resistance.

- Antimicrobial stewardship (AMS) programs aim to slow the development of antimicrobial resistance through judicious, monitored use of antibiotics.

- Traditionally, AMS programs have included pharmacists, physicians, and other healthcare professionals. Registered nurses have been excluded from AMP programs.

- Critical care nurses spend extensive time at the patient bedside and already perform numerous nursing tasks with AWS functions.

- The central role of intensive care unit (ICU) nurse-driven interventions includes numerous functions integral to the successful operation of AMS programs.

REFERENCES

1. CDC. About antimicrobial resistance. Centers for Disease Control and Prevention; 2020. Available at: https://www.cdc.gov/drugresistance/about.html. Accessed March 7, 2020.
2. Burnham JP, Olsen MA, Kollef MH. Re-estimating annual deaths due to multidrug-resistant organism infections. Infect Control Hosp Epidemiol 2019;40(1):112–3.

3. Infectious Disease Society of America (IDSA). New estimate of annual deaths caused by treatment resistant infections highlights gaps in research, stewardship, surveillance. 2018. Available at: https://www.idsociety.org/news%5fpublications-new/articles/2018/new-estimate-of-annual-deaths-caused-by-treatment-resistant-infections-highlights-gaps-in-research-stewardship-surveillance/. Accessed March 7, 2020.

4. Centers for Disease Control and Prevention. A public health perspective on anti-microbial resistance diagnostic: meeting summary and opportunities to address challenges. Centers for Disease Control and Prevention; 2016. Available at: https://www.cdc.gov/drugresistance/pdf/cdc-advameddx-ar-diagnostic-meeting-summary.pdf. Accessed March 7, 2020.

5. Luyt CE, Bréchot N, Trouillet JL, et al. Antibiotic stewardship in the intensive care unit. Crit Care 2014;18(5):480.

6. Bouadma L, Luyt CE, Tubach F, et al, PRORATA trial group. Use of procalcitonin to reduce patients' exposure to antibiotics in intensive care units (PRORATA trial): a multicenter randomized controlled trial. Lancet 2010;375(9713):463–74.

7. Olans RN, Olans RD, DeMaria A Jr. The critical role of the staff nurse in antimicrobial stewardship—unrecognized, but already there. Clin Infect Dis 2016; 62(1):84–9.

8. Manning ML, Pfeiffer J, Larson EL. Combating antibiotic resistance: the role of nursing in antibiotic stewardship. Am J Infect Control 2016.

9. Riley M. Introduction of ANA/CDC working group for engaging nurses in antibiotic stewardship: leadership interview. In: Prevention Strategists, 9. Winter: Association for Professionals in Infection Control and Epidemiology (APIC); 2016. p. 50–7.

10. Edwards R, Drumright LN, Kiernan M, et al. Covering more territory to fight resistance: considering nurses' role in antimicrobial stewardship. J Infect Prev 2011; 12:6–10.

11. Friedman ND. Antimicrobial stewardship: the need to cover all bases. Antibiotics 2013;2(3):400–18.

12. Ladenheim D. Antimicrobial stewardship: the role of the nurse. Nurs Stand 2013; 28(6):46–9.

13. Provonost P, Needham D, Berenholt S, et al. An intervention to decrease catheter-related bloodstream infections in the ICU. N Engl J Med 2006;355:2725–32.

14. Rout J, Bryslewicz P. Exploring the role of the ICU nurse in the antimicrobial stewardship team at a private hospital in Kwa Zulu-Natal, South Africa. So Afr J Crit Care 2017;33(2):46–50.

15. Antibiotic/antimicrobial resistance (AR/AMR): biggest threats and data. Centers for Disease Control and Prevention; 2019. Available at: https://www.cdc.gov/drugresistance/biggest_threats.html. Accessed March 7, 2020.

16. Magill SS, Edwards JR, Bamberg W, et al. Emerging infections program healthcare-associated infections and antimicrobial use prevalence survey team. Multistate point-prevalence survey of health care-associated infections. N Engl J Med 2014;370(13):1198–208.

17. Zingg W, Hopkins S, Gayet-Ageron A, et al. Health-care-associated infections in neonates, children, and adolescents: an analysis of paediatric data from the European Centre for Disease Prevention and Control point-prevalence survey. Lancet Infect Dis 2017;17(4):381–9.

18. Dryden M, Johnson AP, Ashiru-Oredope D, et al. Using antibiotics responsibly: right drug, right time, right dose, right duration. J Antimicrob Chemother 2011; 66(11):2441–3.

19. Strich JR, Palmore TN. Preventing transmission of multidrug-resistant pathogens in the intensive care unit. Infect Dis Clin North Am 2017;31(3):535–50.

20. Kollef MH, Micek ST. Antimicrobial stewardship programs: mandatory for all ICUs. Crit Care 2012;16(6):179.

21. Roberts JA, Paul SK, Akova M, et al. DALI: defining antibiotic levels in intensive care unit patients: are current β-lactam antibiotic doses sufficient for critically ill patients? Clin Infect Dis 2014;58(8):1072–83.

22. Antibiotic stewardship Playbook. National Quality Forum; 2015. Available at: https://store.qualityforum.org/collections/antibiotic-stewardship. Accessed March 7, 2020.

23. Fishman N. Antimicrobial stewardship. Am J Med 2006;119(suppl 1):S53–61.

24. Monsees E, Popejoy L, Jackson MA, et al. Integrating staff nurses in antibiotic stewardship: opportunities and barriers. Am J Infect Control 2018;46(7):737–42.

25. Available at:Core elements of hospital antibiotic stewardship programs. Atlanta, GA: US Department of Health and Human Services, CDC; 2014. Centers for disease control and prevention; 2020. Accessed March 7, 2020. http://www.cdc.gov/getsmart/healthcare/implementation/core-elements.html. https://www.cdc.gov/antibiotic-use/core-elements/hospital.html. March 19, 2021.

26. Kullar R, Nagel J, Bleasdale SC. Going for the gold: a description of the Centers of excellence designation by the infectious diseases society of America. Clin Infect Dis 2019;68(10):1777–82.

27. Fact sheet: obama administration releases national action plan to combat antibiotic-resistant. The White House; 2015. Available at: https://www.whitehouse.gov/the-press-office/2015/03/27/fact-sheet-obama-administration-releases-national-action-plan-combat-ant. Accessed March 7, 2020.

28. New Antimicrobial Stewardship Standard. The joint commission. Available at: https://www.jointcommission.org/assets/1/6/New_Antimicrobial_Stewardship_Standard.pdf. Accessed August 21, 2021.

29. 2020 National Patient Safety Goals. The joint commission. National Quality Forum; 2020. Available at: https://www.jointcommission.org/-/media/tjc/documents/standards/national-patient-safety-goals/npsg_chapter_hap_jan2020.pdf.

30. The Joint Commission (TJC). Facts about the reducing of *Clostridium difficile* infections Project. Available at: https://www.centerfortransforminghealthcare.org/improvement-topics/reducing-c-diff-infections/.

31. Olans RD, Nicholas PK, Hanley D, et al. Defining a role for nursing education in staff nurse participation in antimicrobial stewardship. J Contin Educ Nurs 2015; 46(7):318–21.

32. ANA & CDC. Redefining the antibiotic stewardship team: recommendations from the American nurses association/centers for disease control and prevention Workgroup on the role of registered nurses in hospital antibiotic stewardship practices. 2017. Available at: https://www.cdc.gov/antibiotic-use/healthcare/pdfs/ANA-CDC-whitepaper.pdf. Accessed March 7, 2020.

33. Huang SS, Septimus E, Kleinman K, et al. Targeted vs. universal decolonization to prevent ICU infection. N Engl J Med 2013;368:2255–65.

34. Furuya E, Dick A, Prencevich E. Central line bundle implementation in US intensive care units and impact on bloodstream infections. PLoS One 2011;6(1): e15452.

35. Huang S. Catheter-associated urinary tract infections – turning the tide. N Engl J Med 2016;374(22):2168–9.

36. Whitney RB, Avdic E, Carroll K, et al. Gut check: *Clostridium difficile* testing and treatment in the molecular testing era. Infect Control Hosp Epidemiol 2015;36(2): 217–21.
37. Coia JE, Duckworth GJ, Edwards DI, et al. Guidelines for the control and prevention of methicillin-resistant Staphylococcus aureus (MRSA) in healthcare facilities. J Hosp Infect 2006;63(Suppl 1):S1–44.
38. Jeffs L, Law MP, Zahradnik M, et al. Engaging nurses in optimizing antimicrobial use in ICUs: a qualitative study. J Nurs Care Qual 2018;33(2):173–9.
39. Slatore CG, Hansen L, Ganzini, et al. Communication by nurses in the intensive care unit: qualitative analysis of domains of patient-centered care. Am J Crit Care 2012;21(6):410–8.
40. Ha D, Forte MB, Olans R, et al. A multi-disciplinary approach to incorporate bedside nurses into antimicrobial stewardship and infection prevention. Jt Comm J Qual Patient Safe 2019;45(9):600–5.
41. Ha D, Forte M, Broberg V, et al. Bedside nurses improve antimicrobial stewardship and infection prevention outcomes: results of a 3.5-year study in three hospital telemetry units. Open Forum Infect Dis 2019;6(suppl. 2):S704.
42. Dahlin A, Kone V, Skandhan A. CAUTI: a journey of micturition at MICU since 2014. Sixth decennial international conference of healthcare-associated infections. Infect Control Hosp Epidemiol 2020;41(supplement 1):s154–5.
43. Olans RD, Olans RN, Witt D. Good nursing is good stewardship. Am J Nurs 2017; 117(8):58–63.
44. Gracia J, Serrano R, Garrido J. Medication errors and drug knowledge gaps among critical-care nurses: a mixed multi-method study. BMC Health Serv Res 2019;19:640.
45. Manning ML, Giannuzzi D. Keep patient safe: antibiotic resistance and the role of nurse executives in antibiotic stewardship. J Nurs Adm 2015;45(2):67–9.
46. Barlam TF, Cosgrove SE, Abbo LM, et al. Implementing an antibiotic stewardship program: guidelines by the infectious diseases society of America and the society for healthcare Epidemiology of America. Clin Infect Dis 2016;62(10):e51–77.
47. Kollef MH, Bassetti M, Francois B, et al. The intensive care medicine research agenda on multidrugresistant bacteria, antibiotics, and stewardship. Intens Care Med 2017;43(9):1187–97.
48. Olans RD, Hausman NB, Olans RN. Nurses and antimicrobial stewardship: past, present and future. Infect Dis Clin North Am 2020;34(1):67–82.
49. Morris AM, Calderwood MS, Fridkin SK, et al. SHEA white paper: research needs in antibiotic stewardship. Infect Control Hosp Epidemiol 2019;40(12):1334–43.
50. Padigos J, Reid S, Kirby E. Knowledge, perceptions, and experiences of nurses in antimicrobial optimization or stewardship in the intensive care unit. J Hosp Infect 2021;109:10–28.

Pulmonary Infections, Including Ventilator-Associated Pneumonia

Lora Jenkins-Lonidier, DNP, ACNP-BC, FNP-BC, CCRN

KEYWORDS

- Hospital mortality • Pathogens • Hospital-acquired pneumonia (HAP)
- Community-acquired pneumonia (CAP) • Ventilator-associated pneumonia (VAP)
- Pneumonia

KEY POINTS

- Pneumonia is an infection of the lung that can be caused by pathogens, which are viruses, bacteria, or fungi.
- Pneumonia is a financial burden to the health care system ranked among the top 10 expensive conditions, and the most common cause of hospital admissions.
- Community-acquired pneumonia and hospital-acquired pneumonia are identified by the location of attainment of pneumonia.
- Ventilator-associated pneumonia is a lung infection that develops in a patient who is on a ventilator.
- Treatment and management rely on early recognition and implementation of approved regimen.
- Nursing diligence in adherence to strategies to reduce or prevent pneumonia can be an instrumental tool.

INTRODUCTION

Pneumonia is a disease that attacks the young, the old, and the immunocompromised due to their weakness and vulnerability. Approximately 1 to 1.5 million adults seek medical attention and are hospitalized due to pneumonia every year.[1] Close to 50,000 hospitalized individuals die yearly from pneumonia.[1] The Centers of Disease Control and Prevention (CDC) reported that 43,881 deaths occurred in 2019 due to complications related to pneumonia.[1] It is approximated that 50% who develop pneumonia will have sepsis and septic shock.[2] Pneumonias caused by bacteria can be effectively treated with antibiotics, but with antibiotic resistance growing due to overuse and misuse of antibiotics, there is a demand for new antibiotics. With that being said, the death rate due to pneumonia has remained essentially unchanged over the

Administrative NP, Jackson Pulmonary Associates, Jackson, 971 Lakeland Drive, Suite 1052, Jackson, MS 39216, USA
E-mail address: weljlonidier@comcast.net

Crit Care Nurs Clin N Am 33 (2021) 381–393
https://doi.org/10.1016/j.cnc.2021.08.002
0899-5885/21/© 2021 Elsevier Inc. All rights reserved.
ccnursing.theclinics.com

last 50 years.[2] With the persistence in the number of pneumonia admissions every year this can cause a huge burden on the health care systems with cost up to $17 billion for community-acquired pneumonia (CAP).[3,4] Sun and colleagues[5] reported that ventilator-associated pneumonias (VAPs) increase the cost up to $50,000 per episode over CAP.

Pneumonia is the infection of the respiratory systems that involves the lung parenchyma, bronchus, and alveoli caused by bacteria, fungi, and viruses.[6] For this article, treatments are discussed only for bacterial causes. When defining pneumonia common divisions include CAP and nosocomial infections, which include hospital-acquired pneumonia (HAP) and VAP.[7] **Table 1** provides a cataloging on how pneumonia is defined and classification of site. CAP includes individuals who develop pneumonia in the community. Individuals who develop pneumonia in hospitals are distinguished as having HAP. VAP are pneumonias developed while on mechanical ventilation and in the hospital making it part of HAPs. Both HAP and VAP are considered nosocomial infection pneumonias.

COMMUNITY-ACQUIRED PNEUMONIA
Definition

CAP is the acute infectious process of the lungs that occurs in individuals who are not hospitalized and is associated with high morbidity and mortality. The most common causes of CAP are *Streptococcus pneumoniae, Haemophilus influenza, Mycoplasma pneumoniae, Staphylococcus aureus, Legionella species, Chlamydia pneumoniae,* and *Moraxella catarrhalis.*[8,9] The prevalence and environmental exposures of the pathogens vary geographically, affected by risk factors and use of available vaccines and impacted by the season.

Statistics

Statistically the occurrence and morbidity vary depending on the source with Xu and colleagues[10] reporting that CAP is the second most common cause of hospitalization. The report also states the CAP is the most common infectious cause of death. Ramirez and colleagues[11] report that 1.5 million adults are hospitalized annually resulting to 100,000 deaths during these visits. The CDC reported that 3 million individuals were

Table 1	
Pneumonia site classification	
Diagnosis	**Definition**
CAP	Acute infection of the respiratory system acquired outside of the hospital. Includes patients in nursing homes and dialysis units
Nosocomial pneumonia	Incorporates HAP and VAP, with acute infection of the respiratory system acquired in a hospital setting
HAP	Encompasses HAP and VAP that are acquired 48 h or greater after hospital admission
VAP	HAP occurring 48 h or greater after endotracheal intubation
HCAP	A term that did refer to pneumonia acquired in association a health care facility such as following recent hospitalization, nursing home resident, dialysis centers. The term is now obsolete and part of the CAP classification.

Abbreviation: HCAP, health care-associated pneumonia.
Data retrieved and adapted from CDC Statistics, Frantzeskaki and colleagues,[7] and Shebl and Gulick.[17]

diagnosed at emergency room visits with pneumonia with 50,000 dying from complications related to pneumonia.[1]

Risk Factors

Development of CAP increases in individuals aged 65 years or older; in children younger than 5 years; with tobacco, alcohol, and opioid use/abuse; and in the presence of comorbidities such as Congestive Heart Failure (CHF), dysphagia, impaired airway, stroke, malnutrition, diabetes, and lung diseases, including chronic obstructive pulmonary disease, interstitial lung disease, and asthma to name a few.[6] Other at-risk patients are the immunocompromised individuals such as those with human immunodeficiency virus, patient on chronic steroid use, those using chemotherapy/radiation, and recipients of solid-organ transplant. Lifestyle factors including crowded living conditions, low income, and environmental toxin exposure have also increased the risk of CAP.[12]

Clinical Manifestations

CAP clinical manifestations vary depending on the severity of illness in the individual, but the most common complaints include cough, fever, and dyspnea/shortness of breath.[6,8] Pneumonia determined to be severe presents with characteristics of sepsis, sepsis shock, and possibly respiratory distress. Metley and colloegues[9] report that the Infectious Diseases Society of America (IDSA) and the American Thoracic Society (ATS) have developed criteria to determine if pneumonia was considered severe.[9] **Table 2** determines that to be deemed to possess severe CAP the individual must have 1 of the major criteria, which includes respiratory failure on mechanical ventilation or septic shock on vasopressors. In addition, 3 or more minor criteria must be present. These criteria include altered mental status, hypotension, hypothermia, tachypnea, multilobar infiltrates, uremia, leukopenia, thrombocytopenia, or decreased Pao_2/fraction of inspired oxygen ratio.[12]

Table 2
Severe community-acquired pneumonia criteria

Criteria	Components
Major criteria (must fulfill 1)	• Respiratory failure requiring mechanical ventilation • Septic shock requiring vasopressors
criteria (must fulfill 3 or more)	• Confusion or disorientation • Hypotension requiring aggressive fluid resuscitation • Hypothermia (temperature < 36° C) • Respiratory rate $\geq$ 30 breaths/min • Pao_2/Fio_2 ratio $\leq$ 250 • Multilobar infiltrates • Uremia (BUN $\geq$ 20 mg/dL) • Leukopenia (WBC < 4000) without another source • Thrombocytopenia (PLT < 100,000 cells/µL)

Abbreviations: BUN; blood urea nitrogen; Fio_2, fraction of inspired oxygen; PLT, Platelet; WBC, white blood cell.
Data retrieved from Metlay JP, Waterer GW, Long AC, et al. Diagnosis and treatment of adults with community-acquired pneumonia. An official clinical practice guideline of the American Thoracic Society and Infectious Diseases Society of America. Am J Respir Crit Care Med. 2019;200(7):e45–67; and Kalil AC, Metersky ML, Klompas M, et al. Management of adults with hospital-acquired and ventilator-associated pneumonia: 2016 clinical practice guidelines by the infectious diseases Society of America and the American Thoracic Society. Clin Infect Dis 2016;63(5):e61–111.

Treatment/Management

Diagnosing CAP focuses and places emphasis on the clinical manifestations and pulmonary infiltrates noted on chest radiographic and diagnostic testing, including Complete Blood Count (CBC) and Basic Metabolic Panel (BMP). Antibiotic selection for CAP management depends on the severity and drug resistance risk.[13] IDSA/ATS recommendations determine drug selection to include standard regimen, prior methicillin-resistant *Streptococcus aureus* (MRSA), prior *Pseudomonas* infection, recent hospitalization receiving parenteral antibiotics for risk factors of MRSA, or recent hospitalization receiving parenteral antibiotics for risk factors of *Pseudomonas*. **Table 3** is a summary of drug choices as deemed by IDSA/ATS.[9] Nonsevere CAP includes standard regimen of β-lactam plus macrolide or fluoroquinolone. Prior MRSA respiratory isolation obtains standard regimen and adds MRSA coverage; prior respiratory isolation for *Pseudomonas* gets additional coverage for *Pseudomonas* to standard regimen except change in β-lactam drug choice. For patients recently hospitalized and treated for MRSA rapid polymerase chain reaction should be checked and MRSA coverage should be started if positive. For *Pseudomonas*, cultures are recommended and treatment should be implemented only if positive.[9]

Prevention

Education is the key to prevention of CAP. Vaccines such as the influenza, pertussis, and pneumococcal vaccines are available to decrease the risk of bacterial and viral pneumonia and patients should be encouraged to receive them from their primary care physician or while hospitalized.[1] Basic healthy living practices continue to help decrease the risk of pneumonia including receiving flu vaccine each year, hand washing, avoiding being exposed to a person with respiratory infection, smoking cessation, covering mouth/nose while coughing or sneezing to protect others, and ultimately practicing self-care including care of health and medical conditions.[1]

Nursing role is critical in the care of the patient diagnosed with CAP. Interventions include education of disease, the mechanisms of spreading pneumonia, pneumonia prevention methods, available vaccines, and care of comorbidities. During care nursing management includes nursing assessment, including the respiratory system, clinical findings, laboratory findings, and any changes in status. During the assessment, the nurse assesses specifically in the elderly changes in mental status, dehydration, and unusual behavior. Signs of pneumonia should be recognized, and new developments should be reported to appropriate individuals. Nursing priorities are to maintain and improve respiratory function, prevent complications, and provide education.[14]

Clinical Pearls of Community-Acquired Pneumonia

- CAP accounts for 1.5 million hospitalization admissions.
- *S pneumoniae* is the most common cause of CAP.
- Initial antibiotic selection for patients admitted for nonsevere CAP includes monotherapy, respiratory fluoroquinolone, or β-lactam plus macrolide.
- For patients with severe CAP the antibiotic selection is β-lactam plus macrolide or β-lactam plus respiratory fluoroquinolone.

NOSOCOMIAL PNEUMONIA

The occurrence of nosocomial infections has become an increasing danger to hospitalized patients due to the complications that come from prolonged hospitalization and occurrence of multiple organ dysfunction both leading to increased hospital

Table 3
Community-acquired pneumonia severity and drug resistance risk treatment

CAP Severity Classification	Standard Regimen	MRSA Coverage	*Pseudomonas* Coverage
Nonsevere	Fluoroquinolone: Monotherapy: or β-lactam plus macrolide *Fluoroquinolone options:* Levofloxacin (Levaquin) Moxifloxacin (Avelox) *β-Lactam options:* Ampicillin-sulbactam (Unasyn) Cefotaxime (Claforan) Ceftriaxone (Rocephin) Ceftaroline (Teflaro) *Macrolide options:* Azithromycin (Zithromax) Clarithromycin (Biaxin)	If prior isolation of MRSA add: Vancomycin (Vancocin) or linezolid (Zyvox) If recent hospitalization, receiving treatment IV antibiotics for MRSA, suggestion is to obtain rapid nasal PCR and if positive add MRSA coverage while awaiting cultures	If prior isolation of *Pseudomonas* continue standard regimen but exchange to one of the following antipseudomonal β-lactams: Piperacillin-tazobactam (Zosyn) Cefepime (Maxipime) Ceftazidime (Fortaz) Imipenem (Primaxin) Meropenem (Merrem) Aztreonam (Azactam) If recent hospitalization, received IV antibiotics for *Pseudomonas* then implement treatment if cultures positive
Severe	β-Lactam plus macrolide or beta-lactam plus respiratory fluoroquinolone *β-Lactam options:* Ampicillin-sulbactam (Unasyn) Cefotaxime (Claforan) Ceftriaxone (Rocephin) Ceftaroline (Teflaro) *Macrolide options:* Azithromycin (Zithromax) Clarithromycin (Biaxin) *Fluoroquinolone options:* Levofloxacin (Levaquin) Moxifloxacin (Avelox)	If prior isolation of MRSA or recent hospitalization receiving IV antibiotics for MRSA, add coverage Vancomycin (Vancocin) Or Linezolid (Zyvox)	If prior isolation of *Pseudomonas* or recent hospitalization receiving IV antibiotics for *Pseudomonas* switch β-lactam to one of the following antipseudomonal β-lactams: Piperacillin-tazobactam (Zosyn) Cefepime (Maxipime) Ceftazidime (Fortaz) Imipenem (Primaxin) Meropenem (Merrem) Aztreonam (Azactam)

Abbreviations: IV, intravenous; PCR, polymerase chain reaction.
Data extracted from Metlay JP, Waterer GW, Long AC, et al. Diagnosis and treatment of adults with community-acquired pneumonia. An official clinical practice guideline of the American Thoracic Society and Infectious Diseases Society of America. Am J Respir Crit Care Med. 2019;200(7):e45–67; and Torres A, Niederman MS, Chastre J, et al. Summary of the international clinical guidelines for the management of hospital-acquired and ventilator-acquired pneumonia. ERJ Open Res. 2018;4(2):00028–02018.)

mortality. Despite the advances in health care over a 70-year period the incidence of nosocomial infections continues to be present.[15] Nosocomial pneumonia, also known as HAP, includes VAP.

HOSPITAL-ACQUIRED AND VENTILATOR-ASSOCIATED PNEUMONIA
Definition

HAP is a nosocomial pneumonia that is an acute infection of the pulmonary parenchyma that occurs when the patient has been hospitalized for greater than 48 hours.[16] VAP is an element of HAP that occurs in the intensive care units (ICUs) in association of intubation. VAP that occurs within 48 hours of intubation is reported to affect 10% to 20% of mechanically ventilated patients.[17] Despite the advances in critical care with improved antibiotic coverage, supportive care, prevention, and standard of care bundles, HAP and VAP are significantly related to morbidity and mortality.[16] The common pathogens related to HAP and VAP are the gram-negative bacilli that include *Escherichia coli*, *Klebsiella pneumoniae*, *Enterobacter*, *Pseudomonas aeruginosa*, and *Acinetobacter*. Other pathogens causing HAP and VAP are the gram-positive cocci species, including *Staphylococcus aureus*, MRSA, and *Streptococcus*.[18] There is an increasing frequency of multidrug resistant pathogens and pulmonary microbiome linked to HAP/VAP.[19]

Statistics

There is wide variance in statistical data with HAP occurring in 12% to 29% of patients in the ICU. Of the HAPs in ICU, 90% are VAPs. HAPs are the second common infection and leading cause of death of all hospital-acquired infections with mortality of 25% to 50%. The mortality for VAPs is high ranging from 27% to 76%, varying due to present comorbidities.[20] HAP/VAPs increase hospital length of stay by 7 to 13 days.[21]

Risk Factors

Factors that increase the prevalence and incidence of nosocomial HAP and VAP are numerous in that risk factors include age, chronic lung disease, aspiration, previous antibiotic exposure, reintubation or prolonged intubation, trauma, muscle relaxants, glucocorticoids, and malnutrition to name a few.[22] Ellison and Donowitz categorized risk factors as patient related, infection control related, or intervention related.[23] **Table 4** helps in distinguishing and identifying risk factors. Numerous factors impact the occurrence of a VAP, but the one main component is the presence of an artificial

Table 4
Hospital-acquired pneumonia/ventilator-associated pneumonia risk factor categories

Patient Related	Infection Control Related	Intervention Related
Elderly (>70 y of age)	Lack of hand hygiene	Chest or abdominal surgery
Severe underlying disease	Lack of glove use	Reintubation or prolonged
Chronic lung disease/COPD	Contaminated equipment	intubation
Malnutrition	Frequent circuit changes	Mechanical ventilation
Coma	Previous antibiotic exposure	Sedation/opioid exposure
Metabolic acidosis		Paralytics
Alcoholism		Muscle relaxants or glucocorticoids
CNS dysfunction		Intracranial pressure monitoring
Chronic renal failure		
Anemia		

Abbreviations: CNS, central nervous system; COPD, chronic obstructive pulmonary disease.
   Retrieved from Klompas M. Risk factors and prevention of hospital-acquired and ventilator-associated pneumonia in adults. Published online February 28, 2021. Accessed March 22, 2021. Available at: https://sso.uptodate.com/contents/risk-factors-and-prevention-of-hospital-acquired-and-ventilator-associated-pneumonia-in-adults; and Wu D, Wu C, Zhang S, et al. Risk factors of ventilator-associated pneumonia in critically III patients. Front Pharmacol 2019;10:482.

airway such as an endotracheal tube or tracheostomy. Although necessary and unavoidable at times, its existence detours the protective mechanisms of the respiratory system.

Clinical Manifestation

Diagnosing HAP/VAP can be challenging. Traditional signs and symptoms include new infiltrates on chest radiographic studies, fever greater than 38.5°C, leukocytosis, and positive sputum or blood cultures.[24,25]

Diagnosing VAP includes the use of airway management with intubation within 48 hours of criteria, which includes new pulmonary infiltrates with 2 associated findings. The associated diagnostic findings include (1) fever of 38°C or higher, (2) purulent endotracheal secretions, and (3) leukocytosis with white blood cell count greater than 12,000/mm³. Other findings include hemoptysis, crackles, rhonchi, worsening hypoxemia, and increased inspiratory pressure on mechanical ventilation.[24,25]

Treatment/Management

Once the diagnosis has been made the recommendation is for empirical treatments to include gram-positive and gram-negative antibiotics for treatment against *Staphylococcus* and *Pseudomonas*. In 2016 the IDSA printed guidelines for HAP and VAP. **Table 5** provides a list of the suggested antibiotics from IDSA guidelines of 2016. In 2017, European guidelines were released. Recommendations included analysis of the respiratory secretions to reduce overuse of antibiotics. The European guidelines reserve empirical treatment of *Pseudomonas* species to reduce antimicrobial resistance. Selection of antibiotics differs depending on if following the 2017 European or the 2016 IDSA/ATS guidelines. The 2017 guidelines treatment was led by the presence of multidrug resistance risk and presence of shock.[26] **Table 6** reveals the empirical selection of antibiotics based on the presence or risk of multidrug-resistant organisms. Practice may vary, but treatment is usually targeted to the suspected organism of the region using local antibiograms.

Table 5
Infectious Diseases Society of America hospital-acquired pneumonia/ventilator-associated pneumonia antibiotic coverage

Gram-Positive Including MRSA Coverage Antibiotics	Gram-Negative Including Antipseudomonal Coverage Antibiotics: β-Lactam	Gram-Negative Including Antipseudomonal Coverage Antibiotics: Non-β-Lactam
Vancomycin OR Linezolid (Zyvox)	Piperacillin-tazobactam (Zosyn) OR Cefepime (Maxipime) OR Ceftazidime (Fortaz, Tazicef) OR Imipenem (Primaxin) Meropenem (Merrem) OR Aztreonam (Azactam)	Ciprofloxacin (Cipro) Levofloxacin (Levaquin) OR Amikacin (Amikin) Gentamicin (Garamycin) Tobramycin (Tobi) OR Colistin (Coly-Mycin M) Polymyxin B (Poly-Rx)

Extracted from Kalil AC, Metersky ML, Klompas M, et al. Management of adults with hospital-acquired and ventilator-associated pneumonia: 2016 clinical practice guidelines by the Infectious Diseases Society of America and the American Thoracic Society. Clin Infect Dis. 2016;63(5):e61–111.

Table 6
European empirical antibiotic selection

HAP/VAP Based on MDR Pathogen and Mortality Risk		
Low MDR pathogen and low (<15%) mortality risk	High MDR pathogen and/or high (greater than 15%) mortality risk	
Monotherapy antibiotic Ertapenem (Invanz)	Absence of septic shock Monotherapy against gram-negative (antibiotic to be >90% effective against gram-negative bacteria) ± MRSA treatment	Presence of septic shock Dual treatment with *Pseudomonas* gram-negative coverage ± MRSA treatment
Ceftriaxone (Rocephin)		
Cefotaxime (Claforan)		
Moxifloxacin (Avelox)		
Levofloxacin (Levaquin)		

Abbreviation: MDR, multidrug resistance.
Retrieved from Torres A, Niederman MS, Chastre J, et al. Summary of the international clinical guidelines for the management of hospital-acquired and ventilator-acquired pneumonia. ERJ Open Res. 2018;4(2):00028–02018.

Prevention

Measures in the prevention of HAP/VAP require awareness of actions that impact the likelihood of occurrence. HAP prevention includes strategies to decrease contamination, colonization, and aspiration.[27] Hand hygiene should be maintained donning gloves and gowns as appropriate to present nosocomial infection spread.[28] Providing oral care in a nonventilated patient decreases the bacterial load found in the oropharynx leading to aspiration.[29] Keeping the head of bed at 30° or more decreases pooling of secretions on increasing aspiration risk.[30] Closed suction catheters and clean suction technique should be used when needed to prevent contamination. Education remains a strong component in HAP occurrence or development of worsening complications. Using and recognizing strategies is a fundamental intervention of nursing to reduce HAP.[31] Patient education on cessation of smoking and self-care regimen including adherence of treatment plans for chronic diseases and available vaccines should be discussed.

VAP infections have been looked at in numerous studies, and measures focus on how to decrease their incidence or prevention. Three key principles are identified in the reduction of VAP infections, the first being staff education. Atashi and colleagues[32] reported that the presence of barriers in the ICUs in regard to VAPs is multifaceted and diverse. The various barriers per critical care nursing perceptions are classified as interrelated personal barriers, environmental barriers, and barriers within the organizational matrix.[32] **Table 7** distinguishes discoveries of how nursing perceives why barriers occur and prevention strategies are not met. Included in this table are 3 main categories and 10 subcategories. By exposing the possible causes, education can be tailored to changes that are needed. To have a successful reduction in VAP practice, education, and reinforcement are prerequisites. Klompas and colleagues[27] advocated the use of strategies in VAP prevention. Staff committed to a program or evidence-based strategies have the means to make it a successful method of VAP prevention.[31,33] Once staff behavioral changes have occurred then 2 other principles of reducing VAP infections can occur by reduction of colonization and evasion of aspiration.[34]

Table 7
Categories and subcategory barriers of ventilator-associated pneumonia prevention

Main Category	Subcategory
Nurses' limited professional competence	Unfavorable professional attitudes
	Limited professional knowledge
	Low job motivation
	Limited professional accountability
Unfavorable environmental conditions	Nonstandard physical structure
	Inadequate or inappropriate equipment
	Heavy workload
Passive human resource management	Staff shortage
	Inadequate staff training
	Ineffective supervision

Retrieved from Atashi V, Yousefi H, Mahjobipoor H, et al. The barriers to the prevention of ventilator-associated pneumonia from the perspective of critical care nurses: a qualitative descriptive study. J Clin Nurs. 2018;27(5–6):e1161–e70.

Because colonization occurs in the oropharynx and gastrointestinal tract, best practices are motivation to reduce colonization, which is the second VAP prevention principle. VAP reduction of colonization methods as seen in **Table 8** reveals best nursing practices and its benefit. These methods include handwashing, oral hygiene, standard suction protocol, close suction system, maintaining a closed circuit, use of condensation traps, and stress ulcer prophylaxis.[35] The 2 measures used historically but lacking supportive research are the use of saline lavage and closed suction system rinse

Table 8
Ventilator-associated pneumonia reduction of colonization methods

Best Nursing Practice	Benefit
Handwashing and PPE use	Basic action used to reduce colonization and nosocomial spread of bacteria
Oral hygiene	The oropharynx is known for the bacterial flora and pathogenic organisms that when the bacterial load is reduced can decrease colonization
Standardized suction protocol	Unit-/hospital-wide protocol that is adopted by all nursing to reduce colonization and lower infection rate with compliance
Closed suction system	When used this provides a barrier from contaminated and colonized bacteria reducing VAP rate. Also reported to reduce respiratory stress and susceptibility
Closed circuit maintenance	Use decreases outside pathogens from contaminating the circuit. According to CDC, the ventilator circuit must be changed only if visibly soiled or malfunctioning.
Closed condensation traps	Containment and use of traps like the closed circuit decreases external contamination and reduces possible airway dump of contaminated colonization collection
Stress ulcer prophylaxis	Increased risk of gastric hemorrhage due to stress while on mechanical ventilation leads to prophylactic agents that decrease the acidity. Unfortunately with change in pH of the stomach colonization and microaspiration can occur

Retrieved from Refs.[1,28,31,32,34]

protocol. Use of this protocol has suggested harm to the patient by dislodgement of bacteria in the Endotracheal tube (ETT) into the lung as well as episodes of desaturations. Another measure to reduce colonization is decontamination of the digestive tract, but it is also controversial and does not reveal change in mortality; this requires administration of topical antibiotics into the mouth and stomach.

The third principle in VAP prevention is reducing or preventing aspiration. Interventions used to prevent the opportunity of aspiration reduce the risk of VAP occurrence. The most significantly successful measures in aspiration prevention include oral hygiene, subglottic suction, minimal tube manipulation and controlled cuff pressure, reverse Trendelenburg (head of bed up) position, use of postpyloric feeding, and early extubation. Oral suctioning and hygiene is used to decrease oral colonization and is widely recognized as a key preventive strategy. Subglottic suction helps in preventing microaspiration as oral secretions pool above the tube cuff.[30] Endotracheal tubes should be monitored for appropriate placement and maintaining the cuff pressure at a recommended minimum of 20 mm/Hg or greater to decrease microaspiration. Knowledge of maintaining the head of the bed at 30° or greater is effective in preventing aspiration. Postpyloric feeding has many advantages, and the best method of providing nutrition is not defined. However, the risk of aspiration is reduced with small bowel feeding. The best prevention of VAP development is early extubation when appropriate. For minimizing the exposure to VAPs increase the possible prevention of VAP can be encouraged by reducing mechanical ventilation use as able and early liberation.[24]

Clinical Pearls of Hospital-Acquired Pneumonia Including Ventilator-Associated Pneumonia

- HAP and its subset VAP need awareness and early interventions with use of bundles and order sets to reduce occurrence.
- Vigilance action by nursing staff is the best measure to reduce VAP, which carries a 30% to 50% mortality rate.
- The 3 strategies to reduce VAP include staff education, implementation of measures to reduce microbial colonization, and prevention of microbial aspiration.
- Compliance with prevention strategies for HAP/VAP improves patient outcomes and reduces mortality.
- Guidelines for treatment are based on 2016 IDSA/ATS or the 2017 European recommendations

DISCUSSION

Pneumonia is a common infection and causes significant morbidity and mortality. The economic burden of pneumonia in the hospital setting can be substantial and varies depending on the type of pneumonia, risk factors/comorbidities, causative pathogen, and occurrence of complications. CAP, HAP, and the subset VAP are common respiratory infections of hospitalizations. Pneumonia is ranked the eighth leading cause of death, the most common cause of death due to infection, and the second most common source of hospital admissions. There is an increased length of stay that increases cost and mortality. Management of pneumonia should start with early recognition, prevention of complications, and appropriate treatment with antibiotic selection based on possible causative species and area antibiogram.

SUMMARY

Pneumonias that require hospitalization continue to have increased mortality and morbidity. The development of VAP is classified as a nosocomial infection that occurs

48 hours following the introduction of the endotracheal tube. VAP mortality is close to 50% and results in increased length of stay, increased ventilator days, development of decubitus, contractures, muscle weakness, and loss. Preventing complications due to pneumonia and specifically development of VAPs is a significant concern. Despite ventilator support and antibiotic therapy, the most substantial intervention and prevention strategies are part of the nursing care. Data indicated that VAP can be preventable through evidence-based practices/strategies known as bundles. VAP bundle adopted the use of elevating the head of bed by 30°, daily sedation holiday with assessment, gastrointestinal prophylaxis, deep vein thrombosis prophylaxis, and routine oral care with chlorhexidine. With the implementation of the VAP bundle some hospitals are obtaining low VAP rates, but other hospitals continue to struggle. As care of the patient is provided by nursing, the nurse has an important role in preventing VAPs, preventing risk factors, and recognizing early symptoms. The nurse is the patient advocate becoming the nurse champion to protect the patient from infection, risk, complication and be aware and adhere to the strategies that prevent VAP.

CLINICS CARE POINTS

- HAP and VAP with its statistically wide range of occurrence and the number of evidence-based practices shown to reduce the occurrence continues to reveal up to 76% in mortality.
- Further research regarding the utilization of saline lavages and close suction system may provide more necessary information in the prevention of HAP/VAPs.

DISCLOSURE

The author has nothing to disclose.

REFERENCES

1. FastStats - pneumonia. National Center for health Statistics. Pneumonia 2019. Available at: https://www.cdc.gov/nchs/fastats/pneumonia.htm. Accessed March 1, 2021.
2. American Thoracic Society. Top 20 pneumonia Facts-2019. Available at: http://www.thoracic.org/patients/patient-resources/resources/top-pneumonia-facts.pdf. Accessed March 25, 2021.
3. Tong S, Amand C, Kieffer A, et al. Trends in healthcare utilization and costs associated with pneumonia in the United States during 2008–2014. BMC Health Serv Res 2018;18(1). https://doi.org/10.1186/s12913-018-3529-4.
4. Divino V, Schranz J, Early M, et al. The annual economic burden among patients hospitalized for community-acquired pneumonia (CAP): a retrospective US cohort study. Curr Med Res Opin 2019;36(1):151–60.
5. Sun D, Moorthy V, Chang S-C, et al. Economic burden of ventilator-associated, hospital-acquired, healthcare-associated and community-acquired pneumonia in the hospital setting. Open Forum Infect Dis 2016;3(suppl_1). https://doi.org/10.1093/ofid/ofw172.1196.
6. Prabhu FR, Sikes AR, Sulapas I. Pulmonary infections. Fam Med 2016;1083–101. https://doi.org/10.1007/978-3-319-04414-9_91.
7. Frantzeskaki F, Orfanos SE. Treating nosocomial pneumonia: what's new. ERJ Open Res 2018;4(2):00058–2018.

8. Baer S, Colombo R. Community-Acquired Pneumonia (CAP): Practice Essentials, Overview, Etiology of Community-Acquired Pneumonia. eMedicine 2019. Available at: https://emedicine.medscape.com/article/234240-overview. Accessed March 21, 2021.

9. Metlay JP, Waterer GW, Long AC, et al. Diagnosis and treatment of adults with community-acquired pneumonia. An official clinical practice guideline of the American Thoracic Society and infectious diseases Society of America. Am J Respir Crit Care Med 2019;200(7):e45–67.

10. Xu J, Murphy S, Kochanek K, et al. Deaths: final data for 2013. Natl Vital Stat Rep 2016;64(2):1–119.

11. Ramirez JA, Wiemken TL, Peyrani P, et al. Adults hospitalized with pneumonia in the United States: incidence, epidemiology, and mortality. Clin Infect Dis 2017; 65(11):1806–12.

12. Aleem MS, Sexton R, Akella J. Pneumonia in an immunocompromised patient. 2020. Available at. https://www.ncbi.nlm.nih.gov/books/NBK557843/. Accessed March 21, 2021.

13. Sucher A, Falor C, Mahin T. Updated clinical practice guidelines for community-acquired pneumonia. US Pharmacist 2020;45(4):16–20.

14. Cook LK, Wulf JA. CE: Community-acquired pneumonia: a review of current diagnostic criteria and management. Am J Nurs 2020;120(12):34–42.

15. Kollef MH, Torres A, Shorr AF, et al. Nosocomial infection. Crit Care Med 2021; 49(2):169–87.

16. Kalil AC, Metersky ML, Klompas M, et al. Management of adults with hospital-acquired and ventilator-associated pneumonia: 2016 clinical practice guidelines by the infectious diseases Society of America and the American Thoracic Society. Clin Infect Dis 2016;63(5):e61–111.

17. Shebl E, Gulick PG. Nosocomial pneumonia. 2020. PubMed. Published. Available at: https://www.ncbi.nlm.nih.gov/books/NBK535441/. Accessed March 12, 2021.

18. Sadigov A, Mamedova I, Mammmadov K. Ventilator-associated pneumonia and in-hospital mortality: which risk factors may predict in-hospital mortality in such patients? J Lung Health Dis 2019;3(4):8–12.

19. Sole ML, Yooseph S, Talbert S, et al. Pulmonary microbiome of patients receiving mechanical ventilation: changes over time. Am J Crit Care 2021;30(2):128–32.

20. Roch A, Thomas G, Hraiech S, et al. Hospital-acquired, healthcare-associated and ventilator-associated pneumonia. Published online. Infect Dis 2017;258–62.e1. https://doi.org/10.1016/b978-0-7020-6285-8.00029-0.

21. Giuliano KK, Baker D, Quinn B. The epidemiology of nonventilator hospital-acquired pneumonia in the United States. Am J Infect Control 2018;46(3):322–7.

22. Klompas M. Risk factors and prevention of hospital-acquired and ventilator-associated pneumonia in adults. Published online February 28, 2021. Available at: https://sso.uptodate.com/contents/risk-factors-and-prevention-of-hospital-acquired-and-ventilator-associated-pneumonia-in-adults. Accessed March 22, 2021.

23. Ellison RT, Donowitz GR. Acute pneumonia. In: Mandell, Douglas, and Bennett's principles and practice of infectious diseases. Saunders 2014;25–8.

24. Papazian L, Klompas M, Luyt C-E. Ventilator-associated pneumonia in adults: a narrative review. Intensive Care Med 2020;46(5):888–906.

25. Wu D, Wu C, Zhang S, et al. Risk factors of ventilator-associated pneumonia in critically Ill patients. Front Pharmacol 2019;10. https://doi.org/10.3389/fphar. 2019.00482.

26. Torres A, Niederman MS, Chastre J, et al. Summary of the international clinical guidelines for the management of hospital-acquired and ventilator-acquired pneumonia. ERJ Open Res 2018;4(2):00028–2018.

27. Klompas M, Branson R, Eichenwald EC, et al. Strategies to prevent ventilator-associated pneumonia in acute care hospitals: 2014 Update. Infect Control Hosp Epidemiol 2014;35(8):915–36.

28. How to Guide : prevent ventilator-associated pneumonia. Institute for healthcare improvement. Published February 2012. Available at: http://www.ihi.org/resources/Pages/Tools/HowtoGuidePreventVAP.aspx. Accessed December 15, 2020.

29. Hua F, Xie H, Worthington HV, et al. Oral hygiene care for critically ill patients to prevent ventilator-associated pneumonia. Published online October 25. Cochrane Database Syst Rev 2016. https://doi.org/10.1002/14651858.cd008367.pub3.

30. Leasure AR, Stirlen J, Lu SH. Prevention of ventilator-associated pneumonia through aspiration of subglottic secretions. Dimens Crit Care Nurs 2012;31(2):102–17.

31. Meehan CD, McKenna C. Preventing hospital-acquired pneumonia: implementing a fundamental nursing skills bundle can reduce risk. Am Nurse J 2020;15(2):16–21.

32. Atashi V, Yousefi H, Mahjobipoor H, et al. The barriers to the prevention of ventilator-associated pneumonia from the perspective of critical care nurses: a qualitative descriptive study. J Clin Nurs 2018;27(5–6):e1161–70.

33. Warren C, Medei MK, Wood B, et al. A nurse-driven oral care protocol to reduce hospital-acquired pneumonia. Am J Nurs 2019;119(2):44–51.

34. Osti C, Wosti D, Pandey B, et al. Ventilator-associated pneumonia and role of nurses in its prevention. J Nepal Med Assoc 2017;56(208):461–8.

35. Chacko R, Rajan A, Lionel P, et al. Oral decontamination techniques and ventilator-associated pneumonia. Br J Nurs 2017;26(11):594–9.

Invasive Fungal Infections Among Immunocompromised Patients in Critical Care Settings
Infection Prevention Risk Mitigation

May Mei-Sheng Riley, MSN, MPH, RN, ACNP, CCRN, CIC, FAPIC[a,b]

KEYWORDS

- Invasive fungal infections • *Aspergillus* species • Mucormycetes • Zygomycetes
- Protective environments (PE) • Aspergillosis • Mucormycosis

KEY POINTS

- Invasive fungal infection (IFI) is a devastating opportunistic infection responsible for life-threatening complications and death among immunocompromised patients.
- Survival rates improve with early diagnosis and early treatment, but mortality rates are high for patients on severe or persistent immunosuppression therapy.
- Risk factors come from both the hosts themselves and the environment. Risk factors from hosts are not modifiable; some environmental factors are modifiable.

INTRODUCTION

Invasive fungal infection (IFI) is a devastating opportunistic infection responsible for life-threatening complications and death among immunocompromised patients. Opportunistic infections are those that develop mainly in immunocompromised hosts. IFIs are a significant cause of mortality and morbidity. The presence of fungal elements in deep tissue biopsy or needle aspirates that is confirmed on culture or histopathological examination can be described as an IFI.[1] Examples of IFI are cutaneous fungal infection, angioinvasive aspergillosis, pulmonary aspergillosis, pulmonary mucormycosis, rhinosinusitis, and rhinocerebral mucormycosis.

The fungi that have pathogenicity to cause IFIs include molds (*Aspergillus* spp, *Fusarium* spp, *Scedosporium prolificans*, *Mucor*, *Rhizopus* and *Rhizomucor absidia*) and yeasts (*Candida* spp, *Cryptococcus* spp).[1,2] *Aspergillus* species are commonly

Funding and financial disclosure: Nothing to disclose.
[a] Providence Saint Joseph Health System, 2700 Dolbeer Street, Eureka, CA 95501, USA;
[b] Stanford Health Care, 300 Pasteur Drive, Room H0105, M/C 5221, Stanford, CA 94305-5623, USA
E-mail addresses: mriley@stanfordhealthcare.org; mayriley@gmail.com

isolated from immunocompromised patients.[2] Many hospital-associated fungal out-breaks have been reported.[3,4]

The typical characteristics of susceptible populations for health care-associated IFIs are hematological malignancies, post–bone marrow transplantation, solid organ transplantation, acquired or inherited immunodeficiencies, immunosuppressive drugs, high-dose steroid therapy, neonates, other malignancies, chronic lung dis-eases, residence in intensive care units, and thoracic surgery.[3,4]

The cause of fungal infection for the immunocompromised patient population, espe-cially for post–hematopoietic stem cell transplant (HSCT) patients, is multifactorial and is closely related to the patient's immune responses. Developing infection prevention remediation strategies for the control and removal of fungal growth is challenging but essential to ensure patient safety and improve outcomes. Critical care nurses must inform themselves to protect their vulnerable critical patient populations.

A fungal mitigation plan requires a multidisciplinary approach. The purpose of this article is to highlight the infection control and risk mitigation plan to prevent fungal in-fections in critical care settings.

EPIDEMIOLOGY

IFIs represent a serious threat for severely immunocompromised patients. Many out-breaks of health care-associated IFI have been reported worldwide.[3,4] A large system-atic review of the literature from 1974 through 2014 found that university hospitals were the most common settings to report hospital-associated IFI cases.[4] Tertiary care hospitals provide the most medically advanced treatments and admit highly sus-ceptible patient populations, which leads to their having more IFIs.[4]

Molds can be isolated from the environment and in nature where they are found in soil, on decaying vegetation, in the air, and, and in water supplies.[5] Many fungal out-breaks are related to construction and renovation in health care settings. The causa-tive pathogens are typically *Aspergillus species* and mucormycetes (previously called zygomycetes), but other fungi have been reported.[4]

Invasive aspergillosis is associated with increased mortality with an overall case fa-tality rate of 58%. Rates ranged from 25% for cutaneous cases to 88% for central ner-vous system or disseminated cases.[4]

Mucormycosis is frequently a life-threatening infection with overall mortality rates for pulmonary mucormycosis ranging from 50% to 70%. However, mortality rates may be as high as 95% for patients with extrathoracic dissemination.[6] Death attribut-able to mucormycosis varies from 50% to 100% by publication.[4,7] In systemic fungal infections, the outcome of the infection depends more on the hosts' risk factors than on the fungal virulence.[1]

CAUSATIVE PATHOGENS

The most common clinical isolates of *Aspergillus* species that are associated with invasive infection include *Aspergillus fumigatus, Aspergillus flavus, Aspergillus terreus,* and *Aspergillus niger.* Other pathogenic species include *Aspergillus nidulans, A. fla-vus,* and *Aspergillus udagawae.*[5]

The most commonly reported culture-confirmed mucormycosis cases are *Rhizopus* spp, *Mucor* spp, *Cunninghamella bertholletiae, Apophysomyces elegans, Lichtheimia (Absidia)* spp, *Saksenaea* spp, and *Rhizomucor pusillus.*[6]

The causative pathogens of fungal infection outbreaks in hospitals are usually *Aspergillus* species, including *A fumigatus, A flavus, A terreus,* and *A niger;*

occasionally mucormycetes, such as *Rhizopus* species, *Mucor indicus,* or *C bertholletiae;* and other fungi such as *Scedosporium* species or *Fusarium* species.[4,5,7]

DIAGNOSIS

Survival rates improve with early diagnosis and early treatment, but mortality rates are high for patients on severe or persistent immunosuppression therapy.[5] The signs and symptoms for IFI are nonspecific and can be masked by the underlying diseases. For high-risk patient populations, fungal infection should be included as a part of the differential diagnosis.

Patient's medical history, symptoms, physical examinations, image studies, and laboratory tests can provide valuable information to health care providers to consider when diagnosing a probable IFI. If IFI in lungs or sinuses is suspected, a specimen of tissue or fluid from the respiratory system should be obtained for laboratory analysis. Lung or sinus computed tomographic scan has proved to be an excellent diagnostic tool.

Fungal culture-based diagnosis is used clinically to establish and confirm the specific diagnosis. Fungal culture with antifungal drug susceptibilities can make the culture-based diagnosis clinically relevant.

For *Aspergillus* species, along with fungal culture, assay of biomarkers such as galactomannan and β-D-glucan and polymerase chain reaction can be used for establishing a probable diagnosis.[5,8]

For mucormycetes, fungal cultures can exhibit poor sensitivity. Mucormycosis is a serious infection. Early diagnosis and early treatment with prescription antifungal medicine is essential to reducing mortality. Diagnosis is typically established when angioinvasive hyphae are observed during microscopic examination of tissue samples.[6] Health care providers should correlate the histopathological findings with the patient's medical history, symptoms, and image studies to make a diagnosis.

TREATMENT
Treatment of Aspergillosis

Voriconazole or isavuconazole is recommended as primary antifungal therapy for most patients infected with *Aspergillus* species.[5,6,8] Liposomal amphotericin B can be used as a primary therapy for those who are unable to tolerate voriconazole or isavuconazole or have contraindication due to drug interactions. Alternative antifungal drug selections for salvage therapy include amphotericin B lipid complex, the echinocandins (caspofungin, micafungin, or anidulafungin), posaconazole, or itraconazole.

Treatment of Mucormycosis

Lipid formulations of amphotericin B, posaconazole, and isavuconazole are the therapeutic choice; these are intravenous (IV) medicines.

Isavuconazole and posaconazole can be prescribed for treatment if patients with mucormycosis are clinically stable; these are orally administered medications.

Fluconazole, voriconazole, and echinocandins are not effective against mucormycosis. Frequently patients with mucormycosis require surgery to surgically dissect the infected tissue.

Antifungal Prophylaxis

For aspergillosis prophylaxis, antifungal prophylaxis with posaconazole or possibly voriconazole is used for high-risk patients. However, health care providers must weigh the risks and benefits of prophylaxis for each individual patient.

For mucormycosis prophylaxis, there is no recommended antifungal prophylaxis regimen.

PATIENT POPULATION AT RISK AND ENVIRONMENTAL RISK FACTORS

Risk factors can be classified as either host risk factors or environmental risk factors.

Host Risk Factors

Risk factors for aspergillosis

Opportunistic infections are those that develop mainly in immunocompromised hosts. The risk factors of susceptible patient populations acquiring IFIs include neutropenia (<500 neutrophils/mL for >10 days), hematological malignancies, bone marrow transplant or HSCT, solid organ transplantation (especially renal and liver), chemotherapy, HIV infection, systemic corticosteroids for more than 7 days, prolonged treatment with corticosteroids (>4 weeks), prolonged stay in intensive care (>7 days), and invasive medical procedures. Other risk factors are malnutrition, major surgery, and severe burns.[1–4]

Aspergillosis develops more frequently in patients who underwent lung transplant.[9] Among the most important of all risk factors is severe (<100 neutrophils/mL) and prolonged (>10 days) neutropenia.[9] Some factors predisposing patients who underwent HSCT to *Aspergillus* infection are patients with unrelated donors, patients with graft-versus-host disease, patients coinfected with cytomegalovirus, and patients who receive prophylactic ganciclovir for long periods.[9]

However, aspergillosis has been increasingly found in immunocompetent patients with severe respiratory viral infections, including influenza.[8] Many recent publications describe severe coronavirus disease 2019 (COVID-19)-associated pulmonary aspergillosis.[10,11] A new observation in patients with COVID-19 is the development of invasive *Aspergillus* superinfections or coinfections.[12,13] Approximately 5% of patients infected with severe acute respiratory syndrome coronavirus-2 experience severe lung damage due to viral replication, the ensuing cytokine storm, and complex inflammatory processes; this can lead to secondary fungal pulmonary infections early after the disease's onset.[12]

Risk factors for mucormycosis

Mucormycosis is primarily acquired when immunocompromised hosts inhale environmental sporangiospores or via direct inoculation when skin integrity is compromised.[6]

The main risk factors for health care-associated mucormycosis are prolonged steroid therapy, high-dose glucocorticoid therapy, solid organ transplant, poorly controlled diabetes mellitus (both type 1 and type 2), prematurity, penetrating trauma, burns, persistent neutropenia, and hematological malignancies.[4,6,14]

Environmental Risk Factors

Molds such as *Aspergillus* species or mucormycetes originate in the environment, both indoor and outdoor. These microorganisms are ubiquitous and can be isolated from air, soil, water, food, animal excreta, and particularly in decaying organic substrates, including bread, fruits, vegetable matter, and some building materials. For immunocompetent persons, inhaling some fungal spores is not harmful. For immunocompromised patients, breathing fungal spores can lead to pulmonary or sinus infection and may even lead to disseminated fungal infection.

Various environmental risk factors can be related to the onset of fungal infections. These risk factors include construction, renovation, excavation, and demolition work in health care settings; lack of high-efficiency air filters in ventilation systems; the use of mold-contaminated construction materials in patient care areas; contaminated food and water; the presence of potted plants in patient care areas; and use of mold-contaminated linens.[9] Exposing patients to any environmental risk factor should be avoided; for high-risk patients, even 1 colony-forming unit/m[3] is sufficient to cause infection.[3]

TRANSMISSION

The mode of fungal transmission of species such as *Aspergillus* or mucormycetes is not person-to-person. To establish infection, fungal spores must survive attacks from mononuclear and polymorphonuclear phagocytes to germinate into hyphae, the angioinvasive form of infection; this is not a typical person-to-person transmission. This first line of defense requires a strong innate immune response that immunocompromised patients do not have.[5,6] Infection can occur by inhalation of fungal spores, percutaneous inoculation in cutaneous or subcutaneous tissue, penetration into the mucosa or tissue, and ingestion of contaminated food or drink leading to gastrointestinal fungal disease.[5,6]

OUTBREAKS IN HEALTH CARE SETTINGS

In some aspergillosis or mucormycosis cases, it is difficult to differentiate health care-acquired from community-acquired fungal infections. The incubation period for aspergillosis and mucormycosis is unclear and likely varies depending on the infectious dose of fungi and the host immune response.[1,4] Most aspergillosis or mucormycosis cases in hospitalized patients are sporadic in nature.[4]

In health care-associated outbreaks, the primary *Aspergillus* infection site is the lower respiratory tract because the transmission route of fungal spores is through air. Surgical site infection and cutaneous infection are also reported in the literature. Health care-associated fungal infection outbreaks are often found to be associated with hospital construction, renovation, excavation, and demolition.[4] Construction can increase the count of aerosol fungal spores. As a result, fungal infections in the respiratory tract, soft tissue, and wounds occur in high-risk patients.[3,4] Health care-associated outbreaks of primary cutaneous aspergillosis and central nervous system aspergillosis linked to the use of contaminated medical devices have also been documented.[8] Contaminated medical supplies can be vehicles for spreading fungal spores.

Contaminated adhesive bandages, wooden tongue depressors, hospital linens, and building construction are implicated in health care-associated mucormycosis outbreaks.[7,8,15] Infection portals of entry for patients with cutaneous mucormycosis include surgery and presence of medical devices or drainage.[7,8] Further investigation is warranted when the infection occurs at catheter insertion sites or under adhesive devices.[7]

INFECTION PREVENTION RISK MITIGATION PLAN

Patient risk factors are not modifiable. Therefore, it is crucial to remediate environmental risk factors to create a safe patient care environment to prevent fungal infection. Complying with the published guidelines and recommendations is of paramount importance for a favorable outcome.

A comprehensive infection prevention risk mitigation plan requires a multidisciplinary approach including the following major components: engineering control, environmental health and safety, hand hygiene, environmental cleaning and disinfection, and care coordination.

Surveillance

Surveillance (meaning case finding), data collection, data analysis, and reporting of findings are essential. Surveillance data can identify cases, drive practice, improve performance, and measure success.

As the incubation of IFI varies, it is critical to review each case and define each health care-associated IFI based on a consistent definition. A health care institution's infection prevention and control and health care epidemiology department should work with hospital epidemiologists and infectious disease physicians to craft the definition.

Engineering Control for Infection Prevention

Engineering control includes a large scope of practice to meet regulations and published guidelines. The infection prevention and control/health care epidemiology department must collaborate with the engineering maintenance department. The main goals for engineering control in ventilation are to contain and to prevent the spread of airborne contaminants in (1) local exhaust ventilation (ie, source control), (2) general facility-wide ventilation, and (3) air cleaning.[16] This article highlights only some key components.

Ventilation requirements for protective environments

Protective environments (PE) should be created based on the guidelines published for hospital room design and ventilation to protect neutropenic patients and post-HSCT patients.[16–19] PE are specialized patient care areas with a positive pressure differential between a room and the adjacent hallway. Combining high-efficiency particulate air (HEPA) filtration, frequent air changes, and minimization of air leakage into the room creates a safe environment for patients who underwent HSCT.

- There should be at least 12 air exchanges per hour ($\geq$12 ACH).
- Central or point-of-use HEPA filters with 99.97% efficiency for removing particles 0.3 μm or more in diameter should be used, and filters should be replaced regularly per manufacturers' recommendations. During construction, filters should be monitored to determine the optimum time for filter replacement.
- Positive air pressure differential of 2.5 Pa or more (ie, 0.01 inches by water gauge) should be maintained between patient rooms and hallways.
- Airflow should be directed so that intake is on one side of the room and exhaust is on the opposite side.
- Rooms housing Hematopoietic cell transplantation (HCT) patients should be well sealed to prevent air entering from outside, because this allows entry of spores and makes it difficult to maintain pressure differential.
- Pressure should be monitored continuously, especially while rooms are in use. Use of monitoring systems that warn when the pressure differential relative to the corridor or anteroom decreases less than 2.5 Pa should be considered.
- Self-closing doors should be used to help maintain pressure differential.
- Installing windows in doors and walls of HCT recipients' rooms allows nursing staff to observe HCT recipients without opening doors.
- Carpeting should not be installed in corridors outside or in rooms with patients who underwent HSCT. Contaminated carpet has been linked to aspergillosis outbreaks among patients who underwent HSCT.
- For immunocompromised patients in PE, time spent outside the room (ie, for diagnostic procedures) should be minimized.
- Severely immunocompromised patients should be instructed to wear a high-efficiency respiratory protection respirator when leaving the PE during dust-generating activities, such as construction and renovation.[20]

- Design and selection of furnishings should focus on creating and maintaining a dust-free environment.
- Flooring and finishes (ie, wall coverings, window shades, and countertops) used in HSCT centers should be scrubbable, nonporous, easily disinfected, and should collect minimal dust.

Construction, renovation, remediation, repair, and demolition

The source of most outbreaks of hospital-associated aspergillosis is related to inter-institutional construction or renovation with failure to contain spread of contaminated dust generated during the project.[16–20] Careful review of each construction project as a team is needed.

- Establish a multidisciplinary team to coordinate demolition, construction, and renovation projects and take proactive preventive measures before projects start.
- Educate the health care and construction staff in immunocompromised patient care areas about risk of airborne infection associated with construction and ways to control the dispersal of fungal spores during construction.
- Include clauses for mandatory adherence to infection control practices in construction contracts; incorporate penalties for not complying and methods to ensure that problems are corrected in a timely manner.
- Monitor surveillance for airborne fungal infections during construction activities to ensure environmental health and safety, especially for immunocompromised patients.
- Before the inception of the project, perform an Infection Control Risk Assessment review to define the scope of the project, the potential exposure risk of susceptible patients, and the need for infection prevention measures, including the need for dust and moisture containment measures.
- Implement infection prevention measures for external demolition and construction activities.[16,18]
    a. Determine if the facility can operate temporarily on recirculated air; if feasible, seal off adjacent air intakes.
    b. If this is not practical, check the low-efficiency (roughing) filter banks frequently and replace as needed to avoid buildup of particulates.
    c. Seal windows and reduce wherever possible other sources of outside air intrusion (eg, open doors in stairwells and corridors), especially in PE areas.
    d. Avoid damaging the underground water distribution system (ie, buried pipes) to water contamination by dust and soil.
- Studies show that allogeneic HSCT recipients should avoid exposure to construction or other dust-laden environments for the first 6 months following HSCT and during the periods of substantial immunosuppression to prevent potential exposure to molds. Researchers also suggest that outpatient HSCT recipients should reroute travel to an outpatient cancer center to avoid or minimize exposure to construction sites.[17,19]

Health care laundry, textiles, and medical supplies

- Hospital linens should be laundered, packaged, transported, distributed, and stored in a manner that keeps them dry and prevents exposure to environmental contaminants.[21]
- At least one on-site inspection of the laundry facility conducted by hospital staff is needed on an annual basis to ensure quality of service.

- HSCT center personnel should monitor surgical and elastic adhesive tape and wound-dressing supplies (opened and unopened) for mold contamination to prevent transmission to patients.[17,19]
- Wound dressings and bandages that are expired, visibly contaminated by debris or moisture, or in damaged packages should be discarded. Only sterile dressings should be used when arm boards are used to support IV lines. Arm boards should be changed frequently.[17,19]
- Catheter site splints made from unsterile tongue depressors inserted into foam tubing have been associated with a fatal outbreak of *Rhizopus* microspores in low-birth-weight infants. Such splints should not be used.[17,19]

Flowers and plants in patient care areas
Most researchers strongly recommend that potted plants and fresh or dried flowers should not be placed in the rooms of hospitalized HSCT recipients, HSCT candidates in conditioning therapy, and immunosuppressed patients because *Aspergillus* species have been isolated from the soil of potted plants and the surface of flowers.[16–18,20]

Environmental cleaning and disinfection

- Ensure all equipment and devices are sterilized, disinfected, cleaned, and maintained using only Environmental Protection Agency (EPA)-registered compounds as directed by established guidelines and manufacturers' recommendations.[16,17]
- Ensure adherence to standard environmental cleaning with an appropriate disinfectant.
- Use barrier protective coverings as appropriate for noncritical equipment surfaces that
  a. are frequently touched with gloved hands during patient care;
  b. are prone to contamination by blood or other bodily substances; or
  c. have surfaces that are difficult to clean, such as computer keyboards.
- Clean HSCT patient care areas more than once a day with special attention to controlling dust. Clean exhaust vents, windowsills, and all horizontal surfaces with cloths and mop heads that have been premoistened with an EPA-registered hospital disinfectant.
- Thorough cleaning during and after any construction activity, including minor renovation projects, is critical.
- Follow proper procedure when using cloths, mops, and cleaning solutions.
  a. Prepare cleaning solutions daily or as needed and replace with fresh solution frequently according to facility policies and procedures.
  b. Replace the mop head as per policy, at the beginning of each day, and after cleaning up large spills of blood or other bodily substances.
  c. Before reuse, clean cloths and mop heads and allow them to dry.
  d. If budgeting permits, consider single-use disposable mop heads and cleaning cloths as an alternative.
- Use appropriate dusting methods for patient care areas designated for immunocompromised patients:
  a. Wet-dust horizontal surfaces daily by moistening a cloth with a small amount of EPA-registered hospital disinfectant.
  b. Avoid dusting methods that disperse dust (eg, feather-dusting).
  c. Close the doors of immunocompromised patients' rooms when vacuuming, waxing, or buffing corridor floors to minimize exposure to airborne dust.
  d. Ensure that all vacuum cleaners used in the HSCT center are fitted with HEPA filters.

- Clean up water leaks and repair them as soon as possible but within 72 hours to prevent mold proliferation in floor and wall coverings, ceiling tiles, and cabinetry in and around all HSCT patient care areas. Remove all wet, absorbent structural items (eg, carpeting, wallboard, and wallpaper) and cloth furnishings if they cannot be easily and thoroughly cleaned and dried within 72 hours (eg, moisture content 20% by moisture meter readings); replace with new material.
- If cleanup and repair are delayed greater than 72 hours after a water leak, assume the involved materials to contain fungi and handle accordingly. Use a moisture meter to detect water penetration of walls whenever possible to guide decision making. If the wall does not have less than 20% moisture content for more than 72 hours after water penetration, remove it.

Patient care coordination

- HSCT center personnel should educate patients regarding the risks of exposure to construction and aerosolization resulting from activities such as vacuuming that could disturb fungal spores.
- A study showed that an IFI outbreak was characterized by a strong association with exposure to the unprotected environment outside the hematology ward during patient transfer. Coordinating care among departments to minimize out-of-room time can reduce exposure risk for immunocompromised patients during transfer.[22]
- A high number of transfers were found to be associated with the presence of neutropenia likely indicating insufficient protection of patients during transport.

SUMMARY

IFIs remain a dangerous source of morbidity and mortality in immunocompromised patients. High-risk patients can contract fungi from the environment, so it is crucial to create a protective patient care environment. Protecting patients from fungal exposure can enhance their clinical outcomes.

As patients contract fungi through various routes, a multidisciplinary approach is needed to successfully contain hospital-onset IFI. Collaboration among multiple departments and experts can ensure compliance with Environment of Care (EOC) standards and protect vulnerable patients.

CLINICS CARE POINTS

- The signs and symptoms for IFI are nonspecific and can be masked by the underlying diseases. For high-risk patient populations, fungal infection should be included as a part of differential diagnosis.

- The mode of fungal transmission of species such as aspergillus or mucormycetes is not person-to-person and so does not require special isolation. To establish infection, fungal spores must survive attacks from mononuclear and polymorphonuclear phagocytes to germinate into hyphae – the angioinvasive form of infection. This first line of defense requires a strong innate immune response that immunocompromised patients do not have.

- It is crucial to remediate environmental risk factors to create a safe patient care environment to prevent fungal infection. Complying with the published guidelines and recommendations is of paramount importance for a favorable outcome.

REFERENCES

1. Ramana KV, Kandi S, Bharatkumar V, et al. Invasive fungal infections: a comprehensive review. Am J Infect Dis Microbiol 2013;1(4):64–9.
2. Badiee P, Hashemizadeh Z. Opportunistic invasive fungal infections: diagnosis & clinical management. Indian J Med Res 2014;139(2):195–204.
3. Vonberg RP, Gastmeier P. Nosocomial aspergillosis in outbreak settings. J Hosp Infect 2006;63:246–54.
4. Kanamori H, Rutala WA, Sickbert-Bennett EE, et al. Review of fungal outbreaks and infection prevention in healthcare settings during construction and renovation. Clin Infect Dis 2015;61(3):433–44.
5. Thompson GP, Patterson TF. Aspergillus species. In: Bennett JE, Dolin R, Blaser MJ, editors. Mandell, Douglas, and Bennett's Principles and practice of infectious diseases. 9th edition. Churchill Livingstone, Elsevier; 2020. p. 3103–3116e3.
6. Kontoyiannis DP, Lewis RE. Agents of mucormycosis and Entomophthoramycosis. In: Bennett JE, et al, editors. Mandell, Douglas, and Bennett's Principles and practice of infectious diseases. 9th edition. Churchill Livingstone, Elsevier; 2020. p. 3117–3130e.
7. Rammaert B, Lanternier F, Zahar JR, et al. Healthcare-associated mucormycosis. Clin Infect Dis 2012;54(suppl 1):S44–54.
8. Fungal diseases. Centers for diseases control and prevention Web site. 2019. Available at: https://www.cdc.gov/fungal/diseases/index.html. Accessed April, 22, 2021.
9. Galimberti R, Torre AC, Baztán MC, et al. Emerging systemic fungal infections. Clin Dermatol 2012;30(6):633–50.
10. Hoenigl M. Invasive fungal disease complicating COVID-19: when it rains it pours. Clin Infect Dis 2020. https://doi.org/10.1093/cid/ciaa1342.
11. Lansbury L, Lim B, Baskaran V, et al. Co-infections in people with COVID-19: a systematic review and meta-analysis. J Infect 2020;81(2):266–75.
12. Fekkar A, Lampros A, Mayaux J, et al. Occurrence of invasive pulmonary fungal infections in patients with severe COVID-19 Admitted to the ICU. Am J Respir Crit Care Med 2021;203(3):307–17.
13. Pemán J, Ruiz-Gaitán A, García-Vidal C, et al. Fungal co-infection in COVID-19 patients: should we be concerned? Rev Iberoam Micol 2020;37(2):41–6.
14. Roden MM, Zaoutis TE, Buchanan WL, et al. Epidemiology and outcome of zygomycosis: a review of 929 reported cases. Clin Infect Dis 2005;41(5):634–53.
15. Duffy J, Harris J, Gade L, et al. Mucormycosis outbreak associated with hospital linens. Pediatr Infect Dis J 2014;33(5):472–6.
16. Sehulster LM, Chinn RYW, Arduino MJ, et al. Guidelines for environmental infection control in health-care facilities. Recommendations from CDC and the healthcare infection control practices Advisory Committee (HICPAC). Chicago IL: American Society for Healthcare Engineering/American Hospital Association; 2004; 2019. Available at: https://www.cdc.gov/infectioncontrol/pdf/guidelines/environmental-guidelines-P.pdf. Accessed April 20, 2021.
17. CDC, infectious disease Society of America, and the American Society of blood and marrow transplantation. Guidelines for preventing opportunistic infections among hematopoietic stem cell transplant recipients. Recommendations of CDC, the infectious disease Society of America, and the American Society of blood and marrow transplantation. October 20, 2000/49(RR10); 1-128. Available

at: https://www.cdc.gov/mmwr/preview/mmwrhtml/rr4910a1.htm. Accessed April 20, 2021.

18. Weber DJ, Peppercorn A, Miller MB, et al. Preventing healthcare-associated Aspergillus infections: a review of recent CDC/HICPAC recommendations. Med Mycol 2009;47S1:S199–209. Available at: https://pubmed.ncbi.nlm.nih.gov/19274596/.

19. Tomblyn M, Chiller T, Einsele H, et al. Guidelines for preventing infectious complications among hematopoietic cell transplant recipients: a global perspective. Bone Marrow Transplant 2009;44(8):453–558.

20. Tablan OC, Anderson LJ, Besser R, et al. CDC.; healthcare infection control practices Advisory Committee. Guidelines for preventing health-care-associated pneumonia, 2003: recommendations of CDC and the healthcare infection control practices Advisory Committee. MMWR Recomm Rep 2004;53(RR-3):1–36.

21. Sehulster LM. Healthcare laundry and Textiles in the United States: review and Commentary on Contemporary infection prevention Issues. Infect Control Hosp Epidemiol 2015;36(9):1073–88.

22. Gayet-Ageron A, Iten A, Delden CV, et al. In-hospital transfer is a risk factor for invasive Filamentous fungal infection among hospitalized patients with hematological malignancies: a Matched case-control study. Infect Control Hosp Epidemiol 2015;36(3):320–8.

Sepsis

Michael H. Ackerman, DNS, RN, FCCM, FNAP[a],*, Thomas Ahrens, PhD, RN[b],
Justin Kelly, MHI, BSN, RN, CCRN, RHIA[c,1], Anne Pontillo, MHI, BSN, RN, CCRN[d]

KEYWORDS

• Sepsis • SIRS • qSOFA • Surviving sepsis • Bundles • Apoptosis

KEY POINTS

- Sepsis can be prevented.
- Sepsis is the body's response to an infection.
- Early identification of sepsis is the key to survival.
- Proper implementation of the bundles has been demonstrated to improve survival.

INTRODUCTION

The Greek word "sepo," meaning "I rot" was first used by the physician Hippocrates 2700 years ago to describe what was believed to be an internal decay-process that happened to unlucky individuals.[1] Despite awareness of sepsis dating back to the ancient Greeks and the advances in supportive measures and technology, each year 1.7 million Americans develop sepsis, and of that, 270,000 die as a result.[2]

It was not until the nineteenth century that physicians began to theorize that rather than originating internally, the decay process was occurring due to an external organism, or germs. As a result of these theories and subsequent discoveries, the first preventative measure was born, handwashing. The medical community continued to struggle to define sepsis, and without clear definitions, additional preventative measures and treatments varied widely and remained largely unreliable.[1]

This article presents an overview of where we have been and where we are going in the recognition and management of sepsis. The evolution of the definitions and sepsis treatment bundles is presented. In addition, a brief overview of the complex pathogenesis of sepsis is discussed.

[a] Masters in Healthcare Innovation Program, The Ohio State University, Columbus, OH, USA; [b] Viven Health, 006 Woodbridge Creek Court, St Louis, MO 63129, USA; [c] OSU Wexner Medical Center - The James, 460 West 10th Avenue, Room C1138, Columbus, OH, 43210, USA; [d] Nursing Education Department, James Cancer Hospital Solove Research Institute, 660 Ackerman Road, 5th Floor/Room 574, Columbus, OH 43202, USA
[1] Present address: 60 East 8th, Avenue Apartment #148 Columbus, OH 43201.
* Corresponding author. 157 Battle Green Drive, Rochester, NY 14624.
E-mail address: ackerman.249@osu.edu

Crit Care Nurs Clin N Am 33 (2021) 407–418
https://doi.org/10.1016/j.cnc.2021.08.003
0899-5885/21/© 2021 Elsevier Inc. All rights reserved.

THE EVOLUTION OF THE DEFINITIONS

In August of 1991, the American College of Chest Physicians (ACCP) and the Society of Critical Care Medicine (SCCM) held the first ACCP/SCCM Consensus Committee meeting, "with the goal of agreeing on a set of definitions that could be applied to patients with sepsis and its sequelae."[3] From this committee, a better understanding of the Sepsis 1 (SEP1) terms sepsis, severe sepsis, septic shock, and systemic inflammatory response syndrome (SIRS) was developed. At the time, SEP 1 was considered the manifestation of 2 or more of the following SIRS criteria: temperature 38°C or more or 36°C or less; heart rate 90 beats per minute or more; respiratory rate 20 breaths per minute or more, or $Paco_2$ 32 mm Hg or less; and white blood cell count 12,000/mm^3 or more, 4000/mm^3 or less, or 10% or more immature (band) forms as a result of a presumed or documented infection. In addition to these terms, the use of severity scoring methods was recommended and implementation guidelines for the testing and use of new therapies were outlined.

These definitions were adjusted in 2001 to include organ dysfunction, but it was not until 2016 that the newest definition, "as life-threatening organ dysfunction caused by a dysregulated host response to infection" was developed. The original SIRS terminology was replaced with more of a focus on organ dysfunction and failure.[4]

In 2016, the Sepsis 3 (SEP3) Workgroup proposed new definitions, sepsis and septic shock. Sepsis refers to life-threatening organ dysfunction caused by a dysregulated host response to infection, and septic shock is defined as lactate levels increasing more than 2 mmol L^{-1} without hypovolemia and initiation of vasopressor treatment to keep mean arterial pressure greater than 65 mm Hg.[5] In addition, organ dysfunction was defined by an increase of 2 or more organ dysfunctions on the sequential organ failure assessment (SOFA) scoring system. The qSOFA (quick SOFA) score was recommended. The qSOFA scoring system includes altered mental status (Glascow Coma Scale < 15), respiratory rate greater than 22, and systolic blood pressure (SBP) less than 100.[5]

There were and are issues with each of the definitions. Many thought that the SIRS criteria were too general and the scoring system created too many false-positives. Although it is true that there were many false-positives, the goal of a scoring system is to capture as many people as possible who may have sepsis. Many believe that the emphasis on qSOFA does not assess potential life-threatening sepsis early enough. The data are clear that early recognition saves lives. So, it remains to be seen as SEP3 rolls out, how effective it will be (**Table 1**).

PATHOGENESIS OF SEPSIS

Over the years we have learned more and more in regard to what triggers sepsis, how the body responds to sepsis, and what role genetics plays in the pathogenesis of sepsis. As stated previously, back in the early 1990s, Roger Bone published a sentinel paper that identified sepsis as a syndrome. Essentially, this syndrome is the body's inflammatory and immune response to a noninfectious (pancreatitis, vasculitis, trauma, and/or burns, etc.) or infectious source (bacterial, viral, fungal, etc.). For the purposes of this article, we focus on the infectious causes. Sepsis response is systemic that starts as a local nidus of infection and then cascades out of control. To make an analogy to music: "the inflammatory/immune response gets turned on, turned up, and somebody rips off the knobs."

The pathogenesis of sepsis can be examined from 3 perspectives: molecular, cellular, and organ.[4] Over the years we have learned more and more in regard to the molecular dysfunction associated with sepsis. The cascade of events that takes

Table 1
Definition of sepsis

Sepsis 1 (1991)[6]	Sepsis 2 (2001)[7]	Sepsis 3 (2016)[8]
SIRS: systemic inflammatory response to a variety of severe clinical insults: Temperature >38°C or <36°C; heart rate > 90 beats per min; respiratory rate > 20 breaths per min or $Paco_2$ <32 mm Hg; and white blood cell count > 12,000/mm^3; <4000/mm^3 or>10% immature (band) forms	Infection: Documented or suspected and some of the following: *General parameters:* fever (core temperature > 38.3°C); hypothermia (core temperature <36°C); heart rate >90 beats per min or >2 SD above the normal value for age; tachypnea: respiratory rate >30 breaths per min; altered mental status; significant edema or positive fluid balance (>20 mL kg^{-1} over 24 h); hyperglycemia (plasma glucose >110 mg dL^{-1} or 7.7 mML^{-1} in the absence of diabetes	Sepsis is a life-threatening organ dysfunction caused by dysregulated host response to infection *Clinical criteria for sepsis:* suspected or documented infection and an acute increase of ≥2 SOFA points The task force considered that positive qSOFA criteria should also prompt consideration of possible infection in patients not previously recognized as infected
Sepsis is a systemic response to infection, manifested by 2 or more of the SIRS criteria as a result of infection	*Inflammatory parameters:* leukocytosis (white blood cell count > 12,000/μL); leukopenia (white blood cell count < 4000 μL); normal white blood cell count with > 10% immature forms; plasma C-reactive protein > 2 SD above the normal value; and plasma procalcitonin > 2 SD above the normal value	qSOFA criteria: altered mental status (GCS score < 15); systolic blood pressure <100 mm Hg; respiratory rate > 22 breaths per min
Severe sepsis: Sepsis associated with organ dysfunction, hypoperfusion, or hypotension; hypoperfusion and perfusion abnormalities may include, but are not limited to, lactic acidosis, oliguria, or an acute alteration in mental status	*Hemodynamic parameters:* arterial hypotension (systolic blood pressure < 90 mm Hg, MAP < 70 mm Hg, or a systolic blood pressure decrease > 40 mm Hg in adults or < 2 SD below normal for age, mixed venous oxygen saturation > 70%, cardiac index >3.5 L min^{-1} m^{-2})	Septic shock is defined as a subset of sepsis in which underlying circulatory and cellular metabolism abnormalities are profound enough to substantially increase mortality
Septic shock: Sepsis induced, with hypotension despite adequate fluid resuscitation along with the presence of perfusion abnormalities that may include, but are not limited to, lactic acidosis, oliguria, or an acute alteration in mental status; patients who are receiving inotropic or vasopressor agents may not be hypotensive at the time that perfusion abnormalities are measured	Organ dysfunction parameters:arterial hypoxemia (Pao_2 Fio_2 < 300); acute oliguria (urine output <0.5 mL kg^{-1} h^{-1} or 45 mM L^{-1} for at least 2 h); creatinine level increase ≥0.5 mg dL^{-1}	Septic shock can be identified with a clinical construct of sepsis with persisting hypotension, requiring vasopressor therapy to elevate MAP ≥ 65 mm Hg and lactate > 2 mmol L^{-1} (18 mg dL^{-1}) despite adequate fluid resuscitation

(continued on next page)

Table 1 (continued)		
Sepsis 1 (1991)[6]	**Sepsis 2 (2001)[7]**	**Sepsis 3 (2016)[8]**
	coagulation abnormalities (international normalized ratio >1.5 or activated partial thromboplastin time > 60 s); ileus (absent bowel sounds); thrombocytopenia (platelet count < 100,000 μL^{-1}); hyperbilirubinemia (plasma total bilirubin > 4 mg dL^{-1} or 70 mmol L^{-1})	
	Tissue perfusion parameters: hyperlactatemia (>3 mmol L^{-1}); decreased capillary refill or mottling	

Abbreviations: Fio_2, fraction of inspired oxygen; GCS, Glasgow Coma Scale; MAP, mean arterial pressure.

From Gyawali B, Ramakrishna K, Dhamoon AS. Sepsis: the evolution in definition, pathophysiology, and management. *SAGE Open Medicine.* 2019;7:2050312119835043. Available at: https://journals.sagepub.com/doi/full/10.1177/2050312119835043; https://doi.org/10.1177/2050312119835043; page 3; reprinted by permission of SAGE Publications, Ltd.

place starts with molecular dysfunction, which leads to cellular dysfunction and ultimately leads to the organ dysfunction observed at the bedside (**Fig. 1**). One of the challenges in the treatment of sepsis is the lack of the ability to detect the early warning signs of sepsis at the molecular and cellular levels. This topic is discussed in more details later in this article.

To truly understand the pathogenesis of sepsis it is important to understand what is happening at the molecular/cellular level. The immune system is composed of an innate system, a system we are born with, and an acquired system. The acquired system, as the name implies, develops in response to pathogenetic stimuli. Simply put, the innate system is made up of macrophages, monocytes, granulocytes, natural killer cells, and dendritic cells. The skin is also part of the innate immune system. Each of these cells plays a unique and complex role in the immune response.[4] The acquired immune system is composed of T cells, B cells, and immunoglobulins. The immediate response to a pathogen is the role of the innate immune system that recognizes something as harmful or not harmful in immunocompetent people. The delayed immune response is the role of the acquired immune system.

At the molecular/cellular level, there is a rapidly shifting cytokine milieu that makes managing this response very challenging. When first presented with the presence of an antigen, the innate cells immediately produce proinflammatory cytokines. An example is the macrophage produces tumor necrosis factor-alpha. This proinflammatory cytokine is responsible for the fever, lactate production, and tachycardia that we observe in sepsis. The innate immune cells have evolved to detect pathogenic markers produced from bacteria, fungus, and viruses. These markers are called

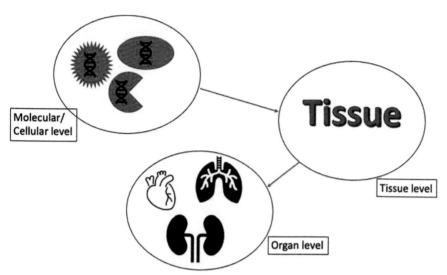

Fig. 1. The progression of sepsis.

pathogen-associated molecular patterns (PAMP) and damage-associated molecular patterns (DAMP).[4] These substances are recognized on the cell surfaces of the innate immune cells by toll-like receptors and other receptors to help defend against the pathogen. In normal amounts, this is an effective defense against the pathogen. However, as stated earlier, if left unchecked, this can lead to the severe reaction seen in patients who are septic. The recognition of PAMP and DAMP stimulate further production of proinflammatory as well as anti-inflammatory cytokines.[4]

In addition to the recognition of PAMP and DAMP by innate immune cells, the complement system, mostly C5a, is activated, which leads to the release of tissue factor, which results in vascular permeability as well as a dysregulation of clotting system. This dysregulation leads to immunothrombosis as well as decreased fibrinolysis, or the ability to break up clot; this has been especially true in coronavirus disease 2019.[6] In addition, there is an upregulation of apoptosis or gene-regulated cell death.

At the tissue and organ levels, the effects of the cellular dysfunction are manifested. The organ dysfunction observed in sepsis is a direct effect of the increased inflammation, immunothrombosis, and impaired fibrinolysis that has gone from a localized response to a systemic response.[7] The vascular permeability observed in sepsis led to the inability to maintain intravascular volume, which then leads to hypoperfusion. Combine that with the myocardial depression observed in sepsis, it is clear to see that left unchecked, this dysregulation is the common pathway of cellular death and ultimately progressive organ failure (**Fig. 2**).

THE EVOLUTION OF THE CARE BUNDLES

In 2001, Rivers and colleagues[8] published a paper that showed that targeting specific goals in resuscitation of the patient with sepsis had a significant improvement in outcome. Before this study, a concern existed that patients with sepsis were being underresuscitated in terms of fluid. In this study, the focus was on using hemodynamic end points to optimize fluid resuscitation (**Fig. 3**). The results of this paper were impressive, with an improvement in mortality from 45% in standard care to 30% in the experimental group where fluid was given to end points such as mixed venous

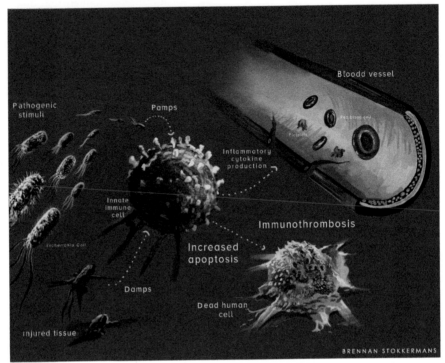

Fig. 2. Sepsis cascade. (*Courtesy of* Brennan Stokkermans, Biology Major, Columbus/Ohio.)

oxyhemoglobin and central venous pressure.[8] The study had some limitations, for example, a single-center study and the use of a specialized team to perform the resuscitation. However, what Rivers and his colleagues[8] accomplished was the beginning of standardized care for the treatment of the patient with sepsis. They used guidelines that were already established by the SCCM. However, they formally studied the criteria in a population of patients with sepsis and are given credit for the first sepsis guidelines and the basis for sepsis bundles.

In 2004, the SCCM and many other major professional societies came together to publish the first recommended treatments for sepsis that would be based on evidence. At this multisociety meeting, which did not include nurses, authors of many of the sepsis papers that were relevant to evidenced-based practice (EBP) were present. Although this session was sponsored by industry, there was no apparent industry influence on the recommendations that came out of this conference. However, just the fact that the conference was sponsored by industry raised concerns over the objectivity of the recommendations.

In 2008, the multisociety meeting was reconvened, this time including nurses.[9] One of the authors of this article (T.A.) was present at this meeting as the representative of the American Association of Critical Care Nurses (AACN). This meeting reflected the need to reconvene regularly to update the guidelines and bundles used in the recognition and management of sepsis. A different system was put into place regarding EBP, for example, the GRADE (Grades of Recommendation, Assessment, Development and Evaluation) system. Also, no industry funding was accepted for this meeting, with all societies funding the representatives. The GRADE system guided assessment

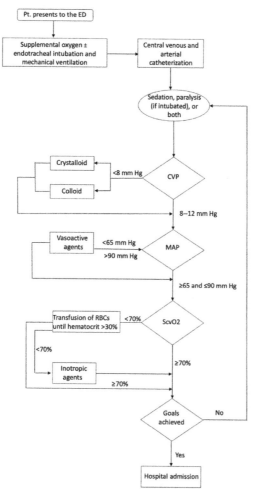

Fig. 3. River's protocol. CVP, central venous pressure; ED, emergency department; Pt., patient; RBCs, red blood cells; ScvO2, mixed venous oxyhemoglobin. (*Adapted from* Rivers E, Nguyen B, Haystad S, Ressler J, Muzzin A, Knoblich B, Petersen E, Tomlanovich M; Early Goal-Directed Therapy Collaborative Group. Early goal-directed therapy in the treatment of severe sepsis and septic shock. N Eng J Med. 2001 Nov 8:345(19) 1368-77. Doi: 10.1056/NEJMoa010307. PMID: 11794169.)

of quality of evidence from high (A) to very low (D) and determined the strength of recommendations. Studies that received a strong or weak recommendation had the following characteristics:

1. Strong recommendation showed that an intervention's positive impact outweighs its undesirable effects (risk, burden, cost) or clearly does not.
2. Weak recommendations indicate that the trade-off between good and bad outcomes is less clear.
3. The grade of strong or weak is of greater clinical importance than a difference in letter level of quality of evidence.

4. Recommendations are grouped into those directly targeting severe sepsis, recommendations targeting general care of the critically ill patient that are considered high priority in severe sepsis, and pediatric considerations.

In 2012, and again in 2016, the evidence-based management of sepsis was reexamined and updated.[10,11] These guidelines addressed many aspects of sepsis management that are important, many that are not directly related to sepsis. As mentioned earlier, some recommendations target general care of the critically ill, for example, proton pump inhibitors for gastrointestinal bleeding and ventilator management guidelines for acute lung injury. This is important because there are no direct treatments for sepsis. However, it is important to have these general care measures to support the patient with sepsis. The bundles helped standardize therapies that may help the patient survive the septic episode. The summary of how the guidelines have progressed over the years can be found in **Fig. 4**.

One should keep in mind that the concept of a bundle is relatively straightforward. This concept is designed to standardized care when managing patients with sepsis. Despite all the attention given to sepsis management from the 2004 to the 2016 Surviving Sepsis Campaign updates, the content in the bundles is simple. The key message with the bundles in terms of sepsis management is to identify patients with sepsis quickly and begin a few treatments rapidly, the faster the better. These recommendations can be seen in the 1-hour sepsis bundle. The Surviving Sepsis Campaign has developed a very nice pocket card that can be found at https://www.sccm.org/getattachment/SurvivingSepsisCampaign/Guidelines/Adult-Patients/Surviving-Sepsis-Campaign-Hour-1-Bundle.pdf?lang=en-US.

CONTROVERSY DUE TO LACK OF INDIVIDUALIZATION

Bundles will come under some criticism because they seem to limit individual treatments and assume that most patients could be treated the same way. Of course, that concept is not accurate and bundle management needs to reflect this lack of

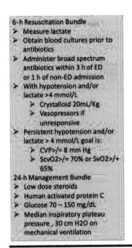

6-h Resuscitation Bundle
➤ Measure lactate
➤ Obtain blood cultures prior to antibiotics
➤ Administer broad spectrum antibiotics within 3 h of ED or 1 h of non-ED admission
➤ With hypotension and/or lactate >4 mmol/L
  ➤ Crystalloid 20mL/Kg
  ➤ Vasopressors if unresponsive
➤ Persistent hypotension and/or lactate > 4 mmol/L goal is:
  ➤ CVP>/= 8 mm Hg
  ➤ ScvO2>/= 70% or SvO2>/+ 65%
24-h Management Bundle
➤ Low dose steroids
➤ Human activated protein C
➤ Glucose 70 – 150 mg/dL
➤ Median inspiratory plateau pressure , 30 cm H2O on mechanical ventilation

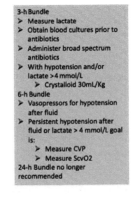

3-h Bundle
➤ Measure lactate
➤ Obtain blood cultures prior to antibiotics
➤ Administer broad spectrum antibiotics
➤ With hypotension and/or lactate >4 mmol/L
  ➤ Crystalloid 30mL/Kg
6-h Bundle
➤ Vasopressors for hypotension after fluid
➤ Persistent hypotension after fluid or lactate > 4 mmol/L goal is:
  ➤ Measure CVP
  ➤ Measure ScvO2
24-h Bundle no longer recommended

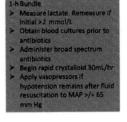

1-h Bundle
➤ Measure lactate. Remeasure if initial >2 mmol/L
➤ Obtain blood cultures prior to antibiotics
➤ Administer broad spectrum antibiotics
➤ Begin rapid crystalloid 30mL/hr
➤ Apply vasopressors if hypotension remains after fluid resuscitation to MAP >/= 65 mm Hg

| 2005 | 2013 | 2018 |

Fig. 4. The history of bundle progression. (*Data from* Refs.[1,3–5,10].)

individualization. Fluid administration is perhaps the most obvious example of the need for individualization. Patients with heart failure or kidney disease often have delicate fluid needs. A bolus dose of 30 mL/kg could potentially make their condition worse.

The recommendation is that the bundles be used as a guide. However, some have mistaken this to mean the bundle needs to be applied to everyone the same way. Governmental bodies such as Centers for Medicare and Medicaid Services will actually financially penalize hospitals if bundle compliance is not rigidly followed. Again, the bundles were designed to act as a guide for all clinicians to use. Compliance with bundles of care is important though, and if exceptions need to be applied, the exceptions need to be carefully explained and documented in the patient's medical records.

Has the use of the sepsis bundles shown improvement in patient outcomes? There are data that suggest this is the case. However, what aspect of the bundle makes the biggest difference? A study by Seymour and colleagues[12] suggests that early antibiotic administration is the key. Other aspects of the bundle such as fluid administration did not seem to play as significant a role. A study by Ferguson and colleagues[13] indicated that a nurse-led sepsis bundle approach improved patient outcomes, including mortality; this was a 7-year study that supports the role of nurses in use of sepsis bundles.

Some government agencies began requiring sepsis bundles with the initial one being New York. In 2013, the New York State Department of Health began a mandatory statewide initiative to improve early recognition and treatment of severe sepsis and septic shock.[14] This was a large initiative reviewing 74,293 (81.3% of patients) patients who had the sepsis protocol initiated. Risk-adjusted mortality decreased from 28.8% to 24.4% ($P < .001$) in patients among whom a sepsis protocol was initiated.[14] Better hospital compliance with the bundles was associated with shorter length of stay and lower risk and reliability-adjusted mortality.

However, the use of bundles has improved the management of patients with sepsis. An interesting example that the bundles have improved the management of patients with sepsis over the past 20 years has been in 3 large studies that were performed in different parts of the world. These 3 studies were the ProCESS (Protocolized Care for Early Septic Shock), ARISE (Australasian Resuscitation in Sepsis Evaluation), and ProMISe (The Protocolized Management in Sepsis) trials.[15–17] These 3 studies asked the question was early goal-directed therapy (EGDT) in regard to fluid resuscitation associated with an improvement in patient outcomes. The studies showed that the early goal-directed guidelines did not seem to make a difference. However, the key thing that was common with all these studies was that they already had performed resuscitation before the EGDT was initiated. In other words, the management of patients with sepsis had been so altered since the 2001 paper by Rivers and colleagues[8] that patients had already been fluid resuscitated.

So, do bundles make a difference in the management of patients with sepsis? The answer would seem to be yes.

THE FUTURE OF SEPSIS RECOGNITION AND THERAPY

When looking at the future of sepsis management, particularly from a nursing perspective, rapid identification of patients with sepsis is necessary. Currently there are no specific tests for sepsis because we have not even been able to define sepsis. Given that sepsis is likely a series of events involving the immune system, different tests are likely to detect different types of septic responses.

Biomarkers

Current tests used to identify sepsis include white blood cell and platelet counts, lactate, and procalcitonin. However, these are nonspecific tests for sepsis. More specific tests that either warn about sepsis or confirm that sepsis is present are needed. For example, genetics will certainly help; one example is a gene expression assay that measures genes associated with one of the key initial responses in sepsis, that is, monocyte distribution width.[18] Monocytes are one of the primary initial defenses against an infection. When they sense an invader, they release a series of cytokines and also become larger. A test like this to evaluate the size of the monocyte is now available and could be available with every white blood cell count. This is the type of early warning sign that is necessary in sepsis identification.

There are many other types of tests that are being developed to improve our accuracy at identifying patients at risk of sepsis or are further down the path with sepsis. It is in this area that in the near future we will be much better at protecting people at risk for sepsis.

Treatments for Sepsis

At present, there is no antisepsis treatment. The most obvious reason that there is no clear treatment of sepsis is that our understanding of sepsis is still limited. We know that sepsis changes from its early stages to multiple organ involvement. It is highly likely that we would need treatments for different stages of sepsis. Roger Bone actually predicted that in the 1990s when he talked about the need for treatment of different stages of sepsis from SIRS to counter anti-inflammatory response syndrome and mixed anti-inflammatory response syndrome.[19] Given this type of varied response in sepsis, and that further individual aspects such as age and genetics are also present, it is difficult to imagine that a single therapy targeting one host mediator will provide benefit to every patient with sepsis. It would make sense based on the aforementioned physiologic situations that there would be personalized medicine for patients with sepsis. For example, instead of every patient getting a certain treatment like a fluid bolus, a therapy would be developed that is targeted to both the patient's genotype and the stage of sepsis. Of course, this is easier said than done. In the near future we would expect to see treatments that are based on targeting specific aspects of the immune system such as antiapoptosis mediators, for example, interleukin-7, a cytokine involved in lymphocyte proliferation and survival.[20] The future for sepsis treatment is wide open but likely to take years before we see specific treatments for sepsis develop.

WRAP-UP

As presented in this article, sepsis and the resulting sequalae of the events that follow is very complex. There is no magic bullet. Our most promising hope is prevention. Although prevention of infection was beyond the scope of this article, great strides have been made in the prevention of infection. As presented, the definitions have evolved over time, as has our understanding of what works and what does not work for treatment. There have been many trials that have failed to show significant effects on morbidity and mortality of sepsis. These are not necessarily failed trials, but trials that have elucidated what will not work and how complex sepsis really is. Finally, the most recent definitions focus on organ function as a screening tool for sepsis, without much discussion of the role of the SIRS criteria. Many feel that this is dangerous. The SIRS criteria still work, and we should do all we can to maintain these criteria as a screening tool until there is something better.

CLINICS CARE POINTS

- Sepsis care bundles reduce morbidity and mortality.
- Early recognition of sepsis is critical to survival.
- Sepsis is a result of the body's response to infection.

DISCLOSURE

The authors have nothing to disclose.

REFERENCES

1. Funk DJ, Parrillo JE MD, et al. Sepsis and septic shock: a history. Crit Care Clin 2009;25(1):83–101. Available at: https://www.clinicalkey.es/playcontent/1-s2.0-S0749070408000808.
2. Centers for Disease Control and Prevention. National center for emerging and Zoonotic infectious diseases (NCEZID), Division of Healthcare quality Promotion (DHQP). Sepsis: clinical information. Centers for disease Control and prevention Web site. 2020. Available at: https://www.cdc.gov/sepsis/clinicaltools/index.html. Accessed June 14, 2021.
3. Bone RC, Balk RA, Cerra FB, et al. Definitions for sepsis and organ failure and guidelines for the use of innovative therapies in sepsis. the ACCP/SCCM consensus conference committee. american college of chest physicians/society of critical care medicine. Chest 1992;101(6):1644–55. Available at: https://proxy. lib.ohio-state.edu/login?url=http://search.ebscohost.com/login.aspx?direct=true&db=rzh&AN=107490724&site=ehost-live.
4. Gyawali B, Ramakrishna K, Dhamoon AS. Sepsis: the evolution in definition, pathophysiology, and management. SAGE Open Med 2019;7. https://doi.org/10. 1177/2050312119835043. 2050312119835043. Available at: https://journals. sagepub.com/doi/full/10.1177/2050312119835043.
5. Singer M, Deutschman CS, Seymour CW, et al. The third international consensus definitions for sepsis and septic shock (sepsis-3). JAMA : J Am Med Assoc 2016; 315(8):801–10. https://doi.org/10.1001/jama.2016.0287. Available at:.
6. Bonaventura A, Vecchié A, Dagna L, et al. Endothelial dysfunction and immunothrombosis as key pathogenic mechanisms in COVID-19. Nat Rev Immunol 2021; 21(5):319–29. Available at: https://www.narcis.nl/publication/RecordID/oai:pure. amc.nl:publications%2Ffe622655-7e64-4444-851d-f4a81815a884.
7. Gotts JE, Matthay MA. Sepsis: pathophysiology and clinical management. BMJ 2016;353:i1585. https://doi.org/10.1136/bmj.i1585. Available at:.
8. Rivers E, Nguyen B, Havstad S, et al. Early goal-directed therapy collaborative group. early goal-directed therapy in the treatment of severe sepsis and septic shock. N Engl J Med 2001;345(19):1368–77.
9. Dellinger RP, Carlet JM, Masur H, et al. Surviving sepsis campaign management guidelines committee. Surviving sepsis campaign guidelines for management of severe sepsis and septic shock. Crit Care Med 2004;32(3):858–73. Erratum in: Crit care med. 2004;32(6):1448. dosage error in article text. Erratum in: Crit care med. 2004;32(10):2169-70. PMID: 15090974.
10. Dellinger RP, Levy MM, Carlet JM, et al. International surviving sepsis campaign guidelines committee; American association of critical-care nurses; American

college of chest physicians; American college of Emergency physicians; Canadian Critical Care Society; European Society of Clinical Microbiology and Infectious Diseases; European society of Intensive care medicine; European respiratory society; international sepsis Forum; Japanese association for acute medicine; Japanese society of Intensive care medicine; society of critical care medicine; society of hospital medicine; Surgical infection society; World Federation of societies of Intensive and critical care medicine. Surviving sepsis campaign: international guidelines for management of severe sepsis and septic shock. Crit Care Med 2008;36(1):296–327. Erratum in: Crit Care Med. 2008 Apr;36(4):1394-6. PMID: 18158437.

11. Dellinger RP, Levy MM, Rhodes A, et al. Surviving sepsis campaign guidelines committee including the pediatric subgroup. surviving sepsis campaign: international guidelines for management of severe sepsis and septic shock: 2012. Crit Care Med 2013;41(2):580–637.

12. Seymour CW, Gesten F, Prescott HC, et al. Time to treatment and mortality during mandated emergency care for sepsis. N Engl J Med 2017;376(23):2235–44.

13. Ferguson A, Coates DE, Osborn S, et al. Early, nurse-directed sepsis care. Am J Nurs 2019;119(1):52–8.

14. Levy MM, Gesten FC, Phillips GS, et al. Mortality changes associated with mandated public Reporting for sepsis. The results of the New York state initiative. Am J Respir Crit Care Med 2018;198(11):1406–12.

15. ProCESS Investigators, Yealy DM, Kellum JA, et al. A randomized trial of protocol-based care for early septic shock. N Engl J Med 2014;370(18):1683–93.

16. Keijzers G, Macdonald SP, Udy AA, et al, ARISE FLUIDS Study Group. The Australasian Resuscitation in Sepsis Evaluation: FLUid or vasopressors in Emergency Department Sepsis, a multicentre observational study (ARISE FLUIDS observational study): rationale, methods and analysis plan. Emerg Med Australas 2019; 31(1):90–6.

17. Mouncey PR, Osborn TM, Power GS, et al. Protocolised Management in Sepsis (ProMISe): a multicentre randomised controlled trial of the clinical effectiveness and cost-effectiveness of early, goal-directed, protocolised resuscitation for emerging septic shock. Health Technol Assess 2015;19(97):1–150, i-xxv.

18. Crouser ED, Parrillo JE, Seymour CW, et al. Monocyte distribution width: a Novel indicator of sepsis-2 and sepsis-3 in high-risk emergency department patients. Crit Care Med 2019;47(8):1018–25.

19. Bone RC. Sir Isaac Newton, sepsis, SIRS, and CARS. Crit Care Med 1996;24(7): 1125–8.

20. Remy KE, Brakenridge SC, Francois B, et al. Immunotherapies for COVID-19: lessons learned from sepsis. Lancet Respir Med 2020;8(10):946–9.

Preventing Central Line Blood Stream Infections in Critical Care Patients

Annemarie Flood, RN, BSN, MPH, CIC, FAPIC

KEYWORDS

- Central line–associated blood stream infections • CLABSI • CLABSI Bundle
- Maintenance bundle

KEY POINTS

- Central line–associated bloodstream infections (CLABSIs) are preventable
- Using a "bundle" approach for both line insertion and line maintenance helps to prevent CLABSI.
- Health care providers need to have training and support to ensure these evidence-based practices are performed.

BACKGROUND

Central lines are intravascular catheters, which end at or near the heart or in one of the great vessels (eg, superior vena cava, brachiocephalic vein, femoral vein).[1] Central lines allow for the provision of care to critically ill patients, deliver nutrition, support renal function, and administer potentially vesicant agents that cannot be administered via peripheral veins.[2] Almost half of the patients admitted to an intensive care unit (ICU) have a central line inserted.[2]

Currently, the Centers for Disease Control reports close to 40,000 central line–associated bloodstream infections (CLABSI) occur in acute care facilities in the United States each year.[1] These events represent 1.4 billion dollars in costs each year and, more importantly, preventable human suffering and death.[3] CLABSI is also a part of Medicare's pay-for-performance (P4P) quality program, "The Hospital-Acquired Condition Reduction Program." Hospitals in the lowest quartile will have payments reduced by 1%, which may have a serious impact on the hospital.[4] The past decade has provided us evidence-based practices that can successfully reduce CLABSI.

Infection Prevention and Quality, City of Hope National Medical Center, 1500 Duarte Road, FLASH Building RM 2219, Duarte, CA 91010, USA
E-mail address: aflood@coh.org
Twitter: @adeluge (A.F.)

Crit Care Nurs Clin N Am 33 (2021) 419–429
https://doi.org/10.1016/j.cnc.2021.08.001
0899-5885/21/© 2021 Elsevier Inc. All rights reserved.

ccnursing.theclinics.com

INSERTION

The Society for Healthcare Epidemiology of America (SHEA) published "Strategies to Prevent Central-Line-Associated Blood Stream Infections in Acute Care Hospitals" in 2008. This document made explicit central line insertion must be considered a sterile procedure, and the document outlines the steps needed to ensure an aseptic technique by implementing maximum sterile barrier precautions.[5] Site choice is important, "wet sites" such as the femoral or jugular vein are associated with a higher infection rate. Therefore, avoid using this site in adults.[5] Lai, Nai Ming, and colleagues[6] found that the use of antimicrobial impregnated catheters was associated with lower catheter-related bloodstream infections (CRBSIs). However, this did not extend to other care settings and did not show any decrease in local site infection, sepsis, or all-cause mortality. However, Yokoe and colleagues[7] do recommend their use in ICU patients.

The insertion procedure should begin with hand hygiene with either soap and water or an alcohol-based hand rub. All personnel involved with the procedure should be wearing a mask, cap, sterile gown, and gloves. The patient should also be completely covered with a large, sterile, fenestrated drape (maximal barrier precautions).[8]

If not contraindicated, the insertion site should be disinfected with a 0.05% chlorhexidine gluconate (CHG)/alcohol solution. One should note that any skin prep used must be allowed to dry naturally and not be blotted or fanned.[8] The catheter should be secured in place by a method other than sutures, as sutures allow for microbial growth. Once the operator has successfully inserted the catheter, a sterile dressing must be applied.[8,9]

Critical care areas should support best practices for the safe and aseptic insertion of central lines. The unit should ensure all the necessary equipment is readily available (eg, having a designated cart with all necessary supplies). The use of a checklist completed by a trained observer is an additional activity that ensures both compliance with maximal barrier use and the maintaining of aseptic technique. Such observers should be given the authority to stop the procedure if there is a break in technique.[8]

Key Takeaways for Insertion

- Use an observer with a checklist of best practices.
- Perform hand hygiene
- Use maximal barrier precautions
- Allow skin preps to air dry completely.
- Place and date a sterile dressing over the insertion site.

MAINTENANCE

For a CLABSI to occur, there must be bacterial colonization of the device. In short-term use (less than 10 days), this colonization most likely occurs when the patient's flora at the insertion site travels along the catheter's outer surface.[10] This knowledge reinforces the need to follow the insertion bundle. The longer a central line remains in place, the more likely hubs and connections will become contaminated if not carefully managed, providing another source of colonization.[10] It is essential that providers practice the techniques appropriately to prevent inadvertent contamination of the central line.

DAILY REVIEW OF NECESSITY

Just as one has more risk of a car accident, the more one drives, the individual patient risk for CLABSI increases as the line is used for more days. A best practice uses a multidisciplinary team to formally review each patient device each day and assess if the patient's condition continues to warrant its use. Patients with multiple devices also have an increased risk of CLABSI. Once the central line is no longer needed for medical care, the best practice is to remove the individual catheters immediately (eg, hemodialysis catheters no longer in use).[5,7,8]

SITE CARE

Health care workers should perform hand hygiene before performing aseptic procedures.

A transparent semipermeable membrane (TSM) dressing is preferred.[5,9] Transparent dressings have several benefits; they allow for visual assessment of the site without dislodging the dressing they prevent moisture. Anchoring the device means less risk of dislodgment or inadvertent removal. They prevent moisture from collecting at the insertion site and can reduce trauma to the skin. After removing the old dressing, disinfect the site with a chlorhexidine-based antiseptic if not contraindicated by age or allergy.[5,9]

In adults, these TSM dressings need changing at least every 7 days. For neonates, central line dressing should only be changed if compromised, soiled, oozing at the insertion site, or there is evidence of compromised skin integrity under the dressing. The use of chlorhexidine-impregnated dressing (eg, chlorhexidine-impregnated sponge or a TSM with chlorhexidine gel) is recommended for adults and children older than 2 months[7,10] who have nontunneled central lines. The use of chlorhexidine in neonates remains unresolved, although many neonatal ICUs have reported its use as part of central line care.[11]

Puig and colleagues[12] found in their recent meta-analysis that using chlorhexidine-containing dressings was effective in reducing CRBSIs in adult ICU patients. If the patient is oozing at the site and does not have a hemostatic dressing or is diaphoretic, use a sterile gauze dressing instead of a TSM and change every 2 days until TSM use is appropriate.[5,9] Only hemodialysis catheters should have antimicrobial ointment applied at the insertion site.[5,9] Any dressing that becomes soiled, dislodged, or wet should be changed regardless of the date it was applied.[5,9] All dressings should be dated after it is applied.[9]

ADMINISTRATION SETS

Tubing changes should be performed aseptically. Pallote and colleagues[13] were able to reduce CLABSI in a neonatal ICU using sterile gloves and placing sterile gauze under the connection point during tubing changes. All connections should be disinfected before the changing of the tubing.[7] Primary and secondary IV tubing sets used for continuous infusion should be changed no sooner than every 96 hours and left in place no longer than every 7 days.[7,9] Tubing should also be changed with the insertion of a new central line.[7,9]

For routine changes of administration sets, consider timing it with the hanging of a new solution bag. Disconnect the patient/open the system as little as possible. If the patient must be disconnected, use a sterile male adapter to protect the tubing with each disconnect.[9]

Change intermittent sets every 24 hours as the repeated connecting and disconnecting offer more opportunities for inadvertent contamination. Tubing should be labeled with the date of the tubing change.[9]

BLOOD, LIPIDS, AND PARENTAL NUTRITION

Administration sets used for blood and blood products should be changed following the manufacturer's instructions for use (IFU). Most sets have a 4-unit capacity.[9]

Because lipids may encourage microbial growth, lipid solution tubing will be changed every 12 hours or with each new container.

Propofol requires changing at least every 12 hours and as frequently as 6 hours, depending on the Instructions for use (IFU).

Parenteral nutrition administration sets must be changed every 24 hours or with every new container, whichever is sooner.[9]

NEEDLELESS CONNECTORS

Needleless connectors protect both the health care worker and the patient. The health care worker is protected from inadvertent needlesticks and the patient from inadvertent disconnection.[14,15] Needleless connectors may be positive, negative, or neutral. There is no advantage of one over the other and staff should follow the IFU for the device used in their institution.[9] They should be changed with the tubing change, not more frequently than 96 hours unless there is residual blood, evidence of contamination, and when the health care worker is drawing blood cultures.[9] A clear connecter may be advantageous for assessing for residual blood or debris.

ACCESSING LINES

Disinfecting the hub or Y site before access prevents the introduction of microbes into the line.[5,7,9] Failures in aseptic technique and disinfection are thought to be the common source of contamination and colonization of central lines.[16] The health care workers, using a disinfectant swab or pad and applying it to the site with mechanical friction for 5- to 15-seconds scrub time, commonly known as "Scrub the Hub," reduces contamination.[9] 70% isopropyl alcohol, iodophors (ie, povidone-iodine), or greater than 0.5% chlorhexidine in alcohol solution are acceptable disinfecting agents.[9]

It is essential to reinforce the hub needs to be scrubbed before each entry into the central venous catheter (CVC). Luckman and colleagues[17] observed that 15 seconds was the most effective length time at removing an externally applied powder; however, the question of what an adequate length of scrub time remains unresolved.[18] The health care worker should follow their institution's policy. A meta-analysis by Flynn and colleagues[18] found using an alcoholic CHG wipe to disinfect the hub was associated with lower rates of CLABSI. Yokoe and colleagues[7] recommended the use of disinfection caps (passive disinfection) on unused ports and y sites to decrease contamination. The use of disinfecting caps in reducing infections was later affirmed by other studies.[18,19] This passive disinfection can assist in reducing contamination of the cap and Y sites. Some caps do not require the user to scrub the hub initially if left in place for a specific time. The health care worker should be familiar with the product's IFU in use in their institution.

PATIENT HYGIENE

Patient hygiene is another important component of CLABSI prevention. There are at least as many bacterial cells on and within the human body as human cells.[20] Coagulase-negative staphylococci, a common skin commensal, is the most prevalent organism reported for CLABSI in the United States.[21] Daily bathing with a CHG solution is recommended for ICU patients.[7] Schier and colleagues,[22] in their study introducing chlorhexidine bathing as a single intervention for ICU patients, saw a 60% reduction in their CLABSI rate. If the patient is capable of showering, protect the dressing and connections from water contamination.[9] Ensure there is adequate staffing to complete patient hygiene and central line care per hospital policy and CDC guidelines.[23] Limit float staff to support standardization of care for unit procedures.[7,21]

Maintenance Take Away

- Assess and remove all unnecessary lines.
- Use a transparent dressing in combination with chlorhexidine when possible.
- Change primary lines no more frequently than every 96 hours.
- Anchor the catheter.
- Date all dressing and tubing changes.
- Use disinfection caps on unused connectors and Y sites
- Scrub the hub.
- Scrub the patient.

SURVEILLANCE

Surveillance is required, not only for a better understanding of a unit's health care–associated infections (HAI) incidence, but also to federal, and in many instances, state reporting requirements.[24] The Center for Medicare and Medicaid requires health care organizations to report their CLABSI surveillance to the National Healthcare Safety Network (NHSN) database. They are required to use the published standard definitions developed by the Centers for Disease Control.[1] A trained infection preventionist should perform this surveillance and provide periodic reports.[1,5]

For surveillance reported to NHSN, a CLABSI occurs when a pathogen grows from one blood culture or a common skin commensal (eg, coagulase-negative staphylococci) grows from 2 closely collected blood cultures and the patient has at least one of the following symptoms: fever (>38.0°C), chills, or hypotension.[21] Also, the patient must either currently have or had (within the last 48 hours) a CVC. The bloodstream infection must not be associated with another infection source (eg, surgical site infection).[21] Events that occur in the first 2 calendar days of admission do not count to the hospital-associated infections. It is a community-associated infection.[21]

It is important to understand that CLABSI is different from CRBSI. The CRBSI definition first requires the same organism to be collected from cultures drawn from both the CVC and a peripheral vein. Then, at least one of the following 3 conditions must occur:

- The bacterial colony count must be at least 3 times higher in the CVC sample.
- The CVC tip culture grows more than 15 colony-forming units of the same organism recovered from the catheter-sourced culture.
- The CVC source culture turns positive at least 2 hours faster than the peripheral source culture.[21]

Practices to reduce CRBSI are usually effective on CLABSI reduction. Considering methods shown to reduce CRBSI can be assessed and added to CLABSI reduction strategies. In addition to surveillance for CLABSI events, we know hand hygiene is the single best way to prevent HAI, not only at the beginning of a procedure like CVC insertion or dressing care but also before each patient encounter. Hand hygiene compliance surveillance and feedback are a necessary part of any HAI reduction program.[25]

EDUCATION

Multiple authorities emphasize the need to have a knowledgeable and competent care team as CVC use is a high-risk activity.[1,5,7,9] The insertion of a CVC and its subsequent care requires multiple steps in specific sequences. Furthermore, without a clear understanding of the evidence underneath the activity, the health care worker is more like to drift away from best practice. Therefore, health care workers need to receive CVC care training when their role first requires it.[1,5,7] They also need to have periodic refresher training after the initial competency and with the introduction of any new technology or products.

Adult learners like health care workers do best with a multimodal approach to education. Including visual and kinesthetic aids in any education presentation for adults leads to increased retention of the material.[25] Educators may find more success with retention if they consider novel approaches to encourage compliance. As an example, one study showed increased compliance with scrubbing the hub for 15 seconds when a musical timer was used rather than education alone.[26]

QUALITY IMPROVEMENT

In 2008, Pronovost[27] published the results of the Keystone Project, where over 100 ICUs in Michigan implemented a CLABSI bundle consisting of a 5-point checklist consisting of:

- Hand hygiene.
- Maximal barrier precautions
- Disinfecting the insertion site with chlorhexidine
- Avoiding femoral sites
- Removing unnecessary CVCs.

This activity successfully reduced CLABSIs by 66% in that state's ICUs.

There have been multiple studies and meta-analyses published since on the successful use of the CLABSI bundle.[28-32] There has also been the development and implementation of a Central Line Maintenance (CLM) bundle.[32-36] The CLM bundle, although not as standardized as the CLABSI bundle, usually includes daily observations of the following:

- Dressing dry, intact, dated, and timed.
- Tubing data and timed.
- Hub disinfection before entry.
- Line necessity review.
- Other elements may include
  - Disinfection caps on all access site
  - Daily CHG bathing.

Synergy occurs when the combination of elements or action produces an effect greater than the sum of its parts. Additional recent examples of bundle success in critical care settings are listed in **Table 1**.

Critical care units that establish standard evidence-based practices, monitor compliance and outcomes, and provide feedback to the individual and the unit have improved outcomes.

UNIT-BASED SAFETY PROGRAMS

One way to operationalize these activities is the introduction of a Comprehensive Unit-Based Safety Program (CUSP). First initiated as part of the Keystone project.[45] and repeated successfully in Rhode Island,[46] CUSP is an 8-step process. It begins with assessing how the staff feels about the organization's commitment to safety. It then moves through education of staff on safety science, identifying safety concerns,

Table 1
Recent examples of bundle success in critical care settings

Author/Year	Type of Study	FOCUS	Outcome	P Value
Richter et al,[37] 2017	Prospective	CLABSI bundle	66% decrease	<.0001
Lin et al,[38] 2018	Prospective	CLABSI bundle	31% decrease	NA
Lai et al,[39] 2018	Prospective	CLABSI bundle	12.2% decrease	<.0001
Arrieta et al,[40] 2019	Prospective	CLABSI bundle	22% decrease	< .01
Gupta et al,[41] 2020	Prospective	CLABSI bundle	0 CLABSI for 3 y	< .05
Russell et al,[42] 2019	Prospective	CLM bundle	61% decrease	.017
Reed et al,[43] 2020	Prospective	CLM bundle	50% decrease	NA
Frith et al,[44] 2020	Prospective	CLM bundle	Improved compliance with bundle	NA

prioritizing, and implementing improvements, and rechecking with staff on their perception of the unit's safety culture after this process.[45] Leadership ownership is a crucial part of a successful CUSP initiative. Higher performing hospitals have leaders who make specific commitments to safety (eg, "zero infections").[47]

CUSP initiatives can be very successful. The Agency for Healthcare Research and Quality and other donors funded "On the CUSP: Stop BSI". More than 100 ICUs across the United States and its territories participated. The program included the development of unit-based multidisciplinary teams, including unit-level and senior-level leadership, front-line staff, and allied and ancillary staff. The overall mean rate for CLABSI dropped from 1.96 to 1.15 per thousand-line days. Almost three-quarters of the participating units reported incident rates of less than one CLABSI for a year and a half after starting the project.[37,46]

HARNESSING THE ELECTRONIC HEALTH CARE RECORD

There is evidence that using an electronic health record (EHR) can reduce adverse patient outcomes.[48] When looking at CLABSI prevention specifically, health care settings may use the EHR to document and trend central line insertion practices, line durations, necessity review, and device day counts.[49] Using these data may help in identifying practitioner and unit-specific opportunities for improvement.

A well-designed EHR can provide asynchronous information about the patient, providing different shifts and care teams information specific to the central line in an efficient fashion. More than 20% of providers in one study did not realize that their patients had a central line.[50] Notifying the team there is a central line and whether or not the line is in active use through an alert or standard workflow can drive review for necessity of use. Other issues could include: if the patient is receiving medication that requires central line use, peripheral venous access issues, or renal replacement (hemodialysis or continuous).[50]

DISCUSSION

The United States has seen a significant reduction in CLABSI since 2008.[1] This reduction happened through using the CLABSI and CLM bundles combined with other practices such as surveillance and user feedback. Public reporting and CMS pay for quality programs also impacted CLABSI reduction. Consistent CLABSI reduction programs require an engaged care team and clear leadership sponsorship, and unit-based resources. Frequent feedback on events and practices keeps the issue front of mind for the team. Optimizing the electronic medical record to enforce activities and improve communication among the team may be the next step in reducing CLABSI. What is clear is CLABSI prevention is a multifactorial process and requires clear goal-setting and ownership by the care team. There is still opportunity for ICUs to provide consistent practice around care bundles.[51-55] It is imperative to remember each CLABSI event means a human being suffered an injury while receiving health care. Health care workers have the accountability to prevent the preventable.

CLINICS CARE POINTS

- Central line insertion and care is a complex high risk, high frequency event in intensive care units, Staff caring for patients with central lines should receive education on central line care before they begin caring for such patients and have their competency assessed on a periodic basis.

DISCLOSURE

The author has nothing to disclose.

REFERENCES

1. NHSN patient safety component manual. National Healthcare safety Network; 2021. Available at: https://www.cdc.gov/nhsn/pdfs/pscmanual/pcsmanual_current.pdf. Accessed March 01, 2021.
2. Milford K, von Delft D, Majola N, et al. Long-term vascular access in differently resourced settings: a review of indications, devices, techniques, and complications. Pediatr Surg Int 2020;36:551–62.
3. Estimating the additional hospital inpatient cost and mortality associated with selected hospital -acquired conditions. Agency for Healthcare Research and Quality; 2017. Available at: https://www.ahrq.gov/hai/pfp/haccost2017-results.html. Accessed March 1, 2021.
4. Hospital-acquired condition reduction (HARCP). Centers for Medicare and Medicaid Services; 2020. Available at: https://www.cms.gov/Medicare/Medicare-Fee-for-Service-Payment/AcuteInpatientPPS/HAC-Reduction-Program. Accessed March 1, 2021.
5. Marschall J, Mermel LA, Fakih M, et al. Society for healthcare Epidemiology of America. Infect Control Hosp Epidemiol 2014;35(7):753–71.
6. Lai NM, Chaiyakunapruk N, Lai NA, et al. Catheter impregnation, coating or bonding for reducing central venous catheter-related infections in adults. Cochrane Database Syst Rev 2016;3(3):CD007878.
7. Yokoe DS, Anderson DJ, Berenholtz SM, et al. A compendium of strategies to prevent healthcare-associated infections in acute care hospitals: 2014 updates. Infect Control Hosp Epidemiol 2014;35(8):967–77.
8. Pronovost P, Needham D, Berenholtz S, et al. An intervention to decrease catheter-related bloodstream infections in the ICU [published correction appears in N Engl J Med. 2007 Jun 21;356(25):2660]. N Engl J Med 2006;355(26):2725–32.

9. Gorski LA, Hadaway L, Hagle ME, et al. Infusion therapy standards of practice, 8th Edition. J Infus Nurs 2021;44(1S Suppl 1):S1–224.

10. Chesshyre E, Goff Z, Bowen A, et al. The prevention, diagnosis and management of central venous line infections in children. J Infect 2015;71(Suppl 1):S59–75.

11. Cho HJ, Cho HK. Central line-associated bloodstream infections in neonates. Korean J Pediatr 2019;62(3):79–84.

12. Puig-Asensio M, et al. Chlorhexidine dressings to prevent catheter-related bloodstream infections: a systematic literature review and meta-analysis. Infect Control Hosp Epidemiol 2020;41(S1):s165–6.

13. Pallotto EK, Piazza JR, Smith TR, et al. Sustaining SLUG Bug CLABSI Reduction: does sterile tubing change technique really work? Pediatrics 2017;140(4): e20163178.

14. Jarvis WR, Murphy C, Hall KK, et al. Health care-associated bloodstream infections associated with negative- or positive-pressure or displacement mechanical valve needleless connectors. Clin Infect Dis 2009;49(12):1821–7.

15. Tarigan LH, et al. Prevention of needle-stick injuries in healthcare facilities: a meta-analysis. Infect Control Hosp Epidemiol 2015;36(7):823–9.

16. Weber DJ, Rutala WA. Central line–associated bloodstream infections: prevention and management. Infect Dis Clin 2011;25(1):77–102.

17. Lockman JL, et al. Scrub the hub! Catheter needleless port decontamination. J Am Soc Anesthesiol 2011;114(4):958.

18. Flynn JM, Larsen EN, Keogh S, et al. Methods for microbial needleless connector decontamination: a systematic review and meta-analysis. Am J Infect Control 2019;47(8):956–62.

19. Barton A. The case for using a disinfecting cap for needlefree connectors. Br J Nurs 2019;28(14):S22–7.

20. Gilbert JA, Blaser MJ, Caporaso JG, et al. Current understanding of the human microbiome. Nat Med 2018;24(4):392–400.

21. Haddadin Y, Annamaraju P, Regunath H. central line associated blood stream infections. [Updated 2020 Dec 14]. In: StatPearls [Internet]. Treasure Island (FL): StatPearls Publishing; 2021. Available at: https://www.ncbi.nlm.nih.gov/books/NBK430891/. Accessed March 12, 2021.

22. Scheier T, Saleschus D, Dunic M, et al. Implementation of daily chlorhexidine bathing in intensive care units for reduction of central line-associated bloodstream infections [published online ahead of print, 2021 Jan 20]. J Hosp Infect 2021;110:26–32.

23. Lee YSH, Stone PW, Pogorzelska-Maziarz M, et al. Differences in work environment for staff as an explanation for variation in central line bundle compliance in intensive care units. Health Care Manage Rev 2018;43(2):138–47.

24. Centers for Disease Control and Prevention. Current HAI progress report. 2020. Available at: https://www.cdc.gov/hai/data/portal/progress-report.html#Tables. Accessed March 14, 2021.

25. Boyce JM, Pittet D. Guideline for hand hygiene in health-care settings: recommendations of the healthcare infection control practices advisory committee and the HICPAC/SHEA/APIC/IDSA hand hygiene task force. Am J Infect Control 2002;30(8):S1–46.

26. Russell SS. An overview of adult-learning processes. Urol Nurs 2006;26(5): 349–52.

27. Caspari L, et al. Human factors related to time-dependent infection control measures: "Scrub the hub" for venous catheters and feeding tubes. Am J Infect Control 2017;45(6):648–51.

28. Pronovost P. Interventions to decrease catheter-related bloodstream infections in the ICU: the keystone intensive care unit project. Am J Infect Control 2008;36(10): S171.e1–5.

29. Furuya EY, Dick AW, Herzig CT, et al. Central line-associated bloodstream infection reduction and bundle compliance in intensive care units: a national study. Infect Control Hosp Epidemiol 2016;37(7):805–10.

30. Latif A, Halim MS, Pronovost PJ. Eliminating infections in the ICU: CLABSI. Curr Infect Dis Rep 2015;17(7):491.

31. Central line associated blood stream infections tool kit and monograph. The Joint Commission; 2017. Available at: https://www.jointcommission.org/resources/patient-safety-topics/infection-prevention-and-control/central-line-associated-bloodstream-infections-toolkit-and-monograph/. Accessed March 3, 2021.

32. Madni T, Eastman AL. Clabsi. In: Salim A, Brown C, Inaba K, et al, editors. Surgical critical care therapy. Cham: Springer; 2018.

33. Padilla Fortunatti CF. Impact of two bundles on central catheter-related bloodstream infection in critically ill patients. Rev Lat Am Enfermagem 2017;25:e2951.

34. Ista E van der Hoven B, Kornelisse RF, et al. Effectiveness of insertion and maintenance bundles to prevent central-line-associated bloodstream infections in critically ill patients of all ages: a systematic review and meta-analysis. Lancet Infect Dis 2016;16(6):724–34.

35. Steele AS, Carlson A, Drummond SL. Diagonal interventions in infection prevention: successful collaboratives to decrease CLABSI at a VA health care system. Infect Control Hosp Epidemiol 2020;41(S1):s191–2.

36. Ben-David D, Vaturi A, Solter E, et al. The association between implementation of second-tier prevention practices and CLABSI incidence: a national survey [published correction appears in Infect Control Hosp Epidemiol. 2019 Nov;40(11):1332]. Infect Control Hosp Epidemiol 2019;40(10):1094–9.

37. Richter JP, McAlearney AS. Targeted implementation of the Comprehensive Unit-Based Safety Program through an assessment of safety culture to minimize central line-associated bloodstream infections. Health Care Manage Rev 2018; 43(1):42–9.

38. Lin WP, Chang YC, Wu UI, et al. Multimodal interventions for bundle implementation to decrease central line-associated bloodstream infections in adult intensive care units in a teaching hospital in Taiwan, 2009-2013. J Microbiol Immunol Infect 2018;51(5):644–51.

39. Lai CC, Cia CT, Chiang HT, et al. Implementation of a national bundle care program to reduce central line-associated bloodstream infections in intensive care units in Taiwan. J Microbiol Immunol Infect 2018;51(5):666–71.

40. Arrieta J, Orrego C, Macchiavello D, et al. 'Adiós Bacteriemias': a multi-country quality improvement collaborative project to reduce the incidence of CLABSI in Latin American ICUs. Int J Qual Health Care 2019;31(9):704–11.

41. Gupta P, Thomas M, Patel A, et al. Bundle approach used to achieve zero central line-associated bloodstream infections in an adult coronary intensive care unit. BMJ Open Qual 2021;10(1):e001200.

42. Russell TA, Fritschel E, Do J, et al. Minimizing central line-associated bloodstream infections in a high-acuity liver transplant intensive care unit. Am J Infect Control 2019;47(3):305–12.

43. Reed E, Mitchell E, Barton K, et al. Multidisciplinary central-line bundle audit Rounding: a strategy to reduce CLABSIs. Infect Control Hosp Epidemiol 2020; 41(S1):s323.

44. Frith J, Hampton D, Pendleton M, et al. Impact of kamishibai card process on compliance with the central venous line maintenance bundle. J Nurs Care Qual 2020;35(1):34–9.

45. Pronovost P, Weast B, Rosenstein B, et al. Implementing and validating a comprehensive unit-based safety program. J Patient Saf March 2005;1(1):33–40.

46. Berenholtz SM, Lubomski LH, Weeks K, et al. Eliminating central line–associated bloodstream infections: a national patient safety imperative. Infect Control Hosp Epidemiol 2014;35(1):56–62.

47. Warrier A, Bernadit S. Impact of leadership walk-arounds and feedback from senior management to reduce CLABSI rates. Infect Control Hosp Epidemiol 2020; 41(S1):s261.

48. Furukawa MF, Eldridge N, Wang Y, et al. Electronic health record adoption and rates of in-hospital adverse events. J Patient Saf 2020;16(2):137–42.

49. Quan KA, Cousins SM, Porter DD, et al. Electronic health record solutions to reduce central line-associated bloodstream infections by enhancing documentation of central line insertion practices, line days, and daily line necessity. Am J Infect Control 2016;44(4):438–43.

50. Thate J, Rossetti SC, McDermott-Levy R, et al. Identifying best practices in electronic health record documentation to support interprofessional communication for the prevention of central line-associated bloodstream infections. Am J Infect Control 2020;48(2):124–31.

51. Burke C, Jakub K, Kellar I. Adherence to the central line bundle in intensive care: an integrative review [published online ahead of print, 2020 Nov 19]. Am J Infect Control 2020. https://doi.org/10.1016/j.ajic.2020.11.014.

52. Scheck A, Hefner JL, Robbins J, et al. Preventing central line-associated bloodstream infections: a qualitative study of management practices. Infect Control Hosp Epidemiol 2015;36(5):557–63.

53. McAlhaney AS, Hefner JL. Getting to zero: goal commitment to reduce blood stream infections. Med Care Res Rev 2016;73(4):458–77.

54. Lee KH, Cho NH, Jeong SJ, et al. Effect of central line bundle compliance on central line-associated bloodstream infections. Yonsei Med J 2018;59(3):376–82.

55. Blot K, Bergs J, Vogelaers D, et al. Prevention of central line-associated bloodstream infections through quality improvement interventions: a systematic review and meta-analysis. Clin Infect Dis 2014;59(1):96–105.

Enlisting Parents to Decrease Hospital-Acquired Central Line–Associated Infections in the Pediatric Intensive Care Unit

Ariel Gilbert, BSN, RN, CCRN*, Cathy C. Cartwright, DNP, RN-BC, PCNS

KEYWORDS

- Central line infections • CLABSI • Hand hygiene • Hospital-acquired infection

KEY POINTS

- Central line–associated bloodstream infections (CLABSIs) are the leading cause of infections in the pediatric intensive care unit (PICU).
- The use of standardized bundles can prevent CLABSIs in the PICU.
- Parents and families should be enlisted to participate in hand hygiene and other central line infection prevention strategies.

INTRODUCTION

Hospital-acquired infections (HAIs), or nosocomial infections, are concerning in all units of the hospital and particularly in the pediatric intensive care unit (PICU). Critically ill children are especially vulnerable to infection due to their immature immune systems and the high volume of providers visiting the patient. Central venous access devices (central lines) are used in pediatric critical care to deliver nutrition, monitoring, and other supportive measures to patients, providing a pathway for infection. Central line–associated bloodstream infections (CLABSIs), contribute to increased mortality, morbidity, and the costs of health care.[1] Goudie and colleagues[2] found a CLABSI cost of $55, 646 and prolonged length of stay of 19 days when compared with non-CLABSI controls. CLABSIs are more commonly found in children than adults[3] and are the leading cause of infections in the PICU.[4] In 2011, Umscheid and colleagues[5] estimated that up to 70% of CLABSIs could be prevented. Although utilization of central line bundle policies has helped to decrease the incidence of CLABSI, more needs to be done,[6] which includes educating and enlisting parents in the battle.

Children's Mercy Kansas City, 2401 Gillham Road, Kansas City, MO 64108, USA
* Corresponding author.
E-mail address: arielgilb@gmail.com

Crit Care Nurs Clin N Am 33 (2021) 431–440
https://doi.org/10.1016/j.cnc.2021.08.004
0899-5885/21/© 2021 Elsevier Inc. All rights reserved.

ccnursing.theclinics.com

BACKGROUND

History has shown that infection control practices can decrease morbidity and mortality in hospitalized patients. Dr Ignaz Semmelweis is known as the father of infection control for his discovery that handwashing could drastically reduce the incidence of postpartum infections (childbirth fever).[7] During that time period, it was believed that disease was spread through bad air.[8] Before the germ theory became widespread, Florence Nightingale observed that crowded and unsanitary conditions contributed to the deaths of hospitalized patients.[8] She believed that hospitals should do the sick no harm and worked to improve conditions in hospitals by implementing basic hygiene and ventilation.[8] Through scrupulous attention to infection prevention practices such as hand hygiene, nutrition, and cleanliness, she increased survival rates from 50% to almost 80%.[9]

CENTRAL LINES

A central line is an intravascular catheter residing in a great vessel or near the heart, used for monitoring, infusion, or withdrawing blood.[10] There are 4 major types of central lines: peripherally inserted central catheter (PICC), non-tunneled centrally inserted venous catheter (CVC) (hemodialysis catheters, Broviacs, etc.,), tunneled centrally inserted venous catheter (commonly referred to by their location- subclavian, femoral line, etc., also hemodialysis catheters), and totally implanted venous port device (ports).[11,12] Although PICCs, ports, and tunneled CVCs are also frequently used in acute care settings, these lines can remain intact for months, allowing patients to be discharged home with the line in place.[11] PICC lines are the longest line due to their peripheral insertion placement and can be used for both short-term and long-term care. Umbilical vein catheters are short-term central lines used in neonates and less commonly used in the PICU.

A CLABSI is defined by the Centers for Disease Control and Prevention's (CDC) National Healthcare Safety Network as a positive blood culture specimen from a patient with a central line present at the time of, or 48 hours before, symptom onset or laboratory confirmation.[10] If the patient has an infection at another site in their body, and the same organism is positive in the blood culture, the blood stream infection is not labeled as a CLABSI. Symptoms for patients younger than 1 year may include apnea, bradycardia, and a temperature less than 36° C or greater than 38°C.[10] Symptoms for any age may include a temperature greater than 38°C, chills, and hypotension.[10]

FACTORS FOR INFECTION

Decreasing nosocomial infections is one of The Joint Commission's Nursing Care Center: 2021 National Patient Safety Goals. The Joint Commission[11] claims nontunneled CVCs are the highest risk for CLABSI. However, recent studies have found that PICC lines have a higher rate of CLABSIs.[13] Factors influencing central line infections include type, anatomic location, duration, number of lumens, and line migration. A 5-year multicenter cohort study with 148 participating PICUs examined the incidence of CLABSIs in 74,196 first placed central lines.[13] CVCs comprised 89% of the central lines placed, whereas PICCs comprised 6%.[13] PICC lines averaged placement of 9.9 days versus 3.79 days for CVCs, and the study found that PICC lines had the highest rate of CLABSIs.[13] CVCs had a greater incidence of infection when placed in the femoral vein (31%) compared with the internal jugular vein (17%); however, anatomic locations of PICC lines did not have a significance for CLABSIs.[13] Patients younger than 5 years of age and PICC lines that have externalized during maintenance care are at higher risk for CLABSI.[14] Type of central line, location of central line place-ment, and duration of the line has a significant risk for infection. Earliest removal of central line devices provides the lowest chance for a bloodstream infection.[13] Because of the rate of PICC line–associated CLABSI, Patel and colleagues[13] do not recommend early removal of a CVC to be replaced with a PICC.

PATHOGENS AND TRANSMISSION

In a prospective time-series design study including 176 United States hospitals report-ing PICU and neonatal intensive care unit CLABSIs over a 5-year period (2013–2018), Hsu and colleagues[1] reported that *Enterococcus* species was responsible for 17% to 23% of PICU CLABSIs. The most frequent other pathogens related to CLABSIs in the PICUs included coagulase-negative staphylococci, *Staphylococcus aureus*, *Entero-bacter cloacae*, yeast, *Klebsiella pneumoniae*, and *Serratia marcescens*.[1] In a 3-year study of 20,390 HAIs from 1003 hospitals investigating pediatric nosocomial patho-gens and antibiotic resistance, Lake and colleagues[15] found that 69% of CLABSIs were HAIs, with 23% identified in PICUs. Coagulase-negative staphylococci (15.6%) and *S aureus* (13.2%) were the primary pathogens responsible for all PICU CLABSIs.[15] Other pathogens responsible included *Enterococcus faecalis* (13%), *K pneumoniae/Klebsiella oxytoca* (10.2%), *Enterobacter* species (8%), and *Pseudo-monas aeruginosa* (4%).[15]

The pathogens causing bacteremia in the studies by Lake and colleagues[15] and Hsu and colleagues[1] are most commonly found on normal flora of the skin, intestines, and mucosa or environmentally in contaminated soil and water (**Table 1**). Direct transmis-sion is spread from the reservoir to the host (the patient) by direct contact or droplet transmission. In the hospital setting, an example of direct contact would be skin to skin contact when a parent hugs the child. Indirect transmission may be from airborne transmission, vectors, and vehicles. Droplet spread in the hospital could be aerosol treatments or speaking in close proximity, sneezing and coughing being the more obvious examples. Of concern for CLABSIs, vehicles may be anything in the patient zone: the central line, intravenous (IV) tubing, and the patient's gown[16] (**Box 1**). The

Table 1	
Common pediatric intensive care unit central line–associated bloodstream infection organisms and sources	
Organism	Common Source
Staphylococcus aureus	Nares[28]
Enterococcus species	Intestinal flora[29]
Coagulase-negative staphylococci	Colonized on human and animal skin and mucosa[30]
Enterobacter cloacae	Intestinal flora[31]
Klebsiella pneumoniae	Human oropharynx and intestines[32]
Yeast	Human skin, mucosa, and intestines[33]
Pseudomonas aeruginosa	Environmental: soil and water contaminate[34]

Data from Hsu HE, Mathew R, Wang R, et al. Health Care-Associated Infections Among Critically Ill Children in the US, 2013 to 2018 [published online ahead of print, 2020 Oct 5]. *JAMA Pediatr.* 2020;e203223. doi:10.1001/jamapediatrics.2020.3223. Lake JG, Weiner LM, Milstone AM, Saiman L, Magill SS See l. Pathogen Distribution and Antimicrobial Resistance Among Pediatric Healthcare-Associated Infections Reported to the National Healthcare Safety Network, 2011 to 2014. *Infect Control Hosp Epidemiol.* 2018; 39 (1): 1 to 11. https://www.ncbi.nlm.nih.gov/pmc/articles/PMC6643994/. doi:10.1017/ice.2017.236.

Box 1
Vehicles for pathogen transmission in patient zone

- Gloves
- Central line/PIV/arterial line
- Endotracheal tube
- IV tubing/adapters
- Linens/gowns
- Bed rails
- Call light
- Monitor and remote
- Monitoring devices and cords

Abbreviation: PIV, Peripheral intravenous line.

Data from World Health Organization & WHO Patient Safety. WHO guidelines on hand hygiene in health care. 2009. Available at: https://www.who.int/publications/i/item/9789241597906. Accessed March 30, 2021.

---

full chain of infection occurs, with visitors being the potential host and portal of exit, transmission via direct or indirect contact, and the central venous line site is the obvious portal of entry to the susceptible host—the patient.[17] The number of surfaces a parent or provider touches on entering the patient's room and before touching a child for an assessment or therapeutic comfort puts the patient at high risk of pathogenic exposure. In an effort to decrease cross-contamination, all individuals entering the room must guarantee a focused conscientious effort on hand hygiene.

HEALTH CARE WORKERS

Patient acuity dictates high traffic volume in the patient's room by health care professionals, and the bedside nurse usually has the most frequent contact with the patient. The number of health care professionals entering the patient room daily could include the primary and consulting physicians, respiratory therapists, specialty or resourcing nurses, patient care assistants, physical therapist/occupational therapists, and environmental services. All staff should be attentive to cross contamination and receptive to feedback regarding their hand hygiene, mindfulness, and prevention of cross-contamination. On entering the patient room, there is an expectation to use hand hygiene practices. Quality improvement initiatives often look at increasing hand hygiene practices before entry. However, once in the patient room, there are numerous opportunities for contamination before touching the patient. Therefore, additional emphasis is placed on hand hygiene directly before patient contact.

HAND HYGIENE

The Joint Commission states decreasing nosocomial (hospital-acquired) infections as one of their Nursing Care Center: 2021 National Patient Safety Goals.[18] Elements of performance to decrease nosocomial infections include complying with the CDC or World Health Organization hand hygiene practices, setting goals for compliance, and improving outcomes based on the goals set.[18] Hand hygiene is the most effective way of preventing the spread of germs, and it is an expectation that health care providers adhere to 5 moments of hand hygiene.[16] These moments include (1) before and (2) after touching the patient, (3) after touching the patient's surroundings, (4) before aseptic techniques, and (5) after exposure to bodily fluids. Hand hygiene before and after patient contact helps prevent introducing colonized microorganisms from the health care area to the patient. Patient surroundings are exposed to their own normal flora and to the normal flora of anyone who has contact with that space. Hand hygiene before aseptic technique is one of the most important factors for reducing CLABSIs and may coincide with other moments of hand hygiene.[16] Frequently, the bedside nurse will reposition the patient, or withdraw the bedsheet, to access the central line. Exposure to bodily fluids with or without gloves requires hand hygiene to reduce the risk of spreading colonized microorganisms to a clean site in the same patient, that is, stool to blood stream, and it protects the health care worker from transmission.[16] Barriers to hand hygiene compliance in the PICU include forgetfulness, time-constraints, emergencies, and distractions in the environment.[19] Distractions can include alarms, conversations, and the caregivers' thoughts, causing lack of focus. Hand hygiene is a simple and essential way for patients and families to be involved in the child's care and, at the same time, decrease bacterial spread. Empowering patients and families to be involved in their care promotes teamwork and self-efficacy.

VISITORS

Visitors, including parents, account for approximately a quarter of traffic entering and exiting patient rooms.[19,20] Education for families on proper hand hygiene is imperative and allows them some control over their child's recovery. Education should emphasize when to perform hand hygiene, how long to wash and dry, and why it is of importance in the hospital, particularly what HAI the child is at highest risk for based on devices present.[16] Education should be tailored to the parents' level of understanding and the ability to process information with return demonstration. Campbell and colleagues[19] studied the benefits of educating families on hand hygiene with a visual tool in a Vietnamese PICU. The visual tool was a fan decorated with text and a symbol of a heart and hands as a reminder to use appropriate hand hygiene. Health care workers taught families the importance of hand hygiene, the 5 moments of hand hygiene, and utilization of the fan. The family was responsible to remind the health care personnel to use hand hygiene or correct their practices if using it incorrectly. Although the health care workers were informed before the study, families reported feelings of embarrassment and lacked courage to speak up, even though they recognized opportunities for improvement. The tool allowed the families to communicate without coming up with the words to confront the health care worker. Nurses and physicians reported feeling embarrassed yet grateful when reminded by families and found the tactic effective. The visual tool was reported to be beneficial in comparison to solely a verbal education.[19]

SAFETY CULTURE

In addition to education, cooperation among health care personnel and the patient and family is needed to decrease the incidence of HAIs. A culture of safety is one that encourages speaking up when errors or near misses occur, a blame-free environment of reporting, and commitment to addressing safety concerns.[21] In a review of 55 articles from 2009 to 2019, Braun and colleagues[21] found a relationship between a safety culture, infection prevention processes, and HAIs. Braun and colleagues[21] concluded that a positive safety culture contributes to the success of infection prevention control, although it may be bidirectional. A positive safety culture lacks blame and is not punitive. Practicing these conversations such as "can I offer you hand sanitizer" or "thank you for the feedback" with a calm, nondefensive tone makes in-the-moment conversations more natural.

MAINTENANCE BUNDLES

Central line bundles are grouped elements to decrease the risk for CLABSI, and Solutions for Patient Safety (SPS) outlines bundles for insertion and maintenance.[22] In the pediatric population, maintenance bundles have a greater role in CLABSI prevention compared with adults.[23] Nurses and families have an impact on CLABSI prevention by their hand hygiene practices, advocacy, patient hygiene, and aseptic techniques. Parents and patients can participate in components of the maintenance bundle by assisting with daily linen changes and chlorhexidine (CHG) wipes (if patient is older than 2 months), notifying the nurses if the dressing becomes soiled or loose, and daily participation in the discussion of the line necessity. Patients should be instructed to report any CLABSI symptoms such as site pain, erythema, chills, and malaise. Nurses should discourage the patient and visitors from touching the central line and tubing, although age and development can pose difficulty in compliance. The patient and parents can assist with adherence to hand hygiene by reminding anyone entering the room, especially before touching the patient and accessing the device. SPS[22] recommends evaluating the necessity and functionality of the central line daily, including the frequency of entries and laboratories. Regular assessments include the integrity of the dressing and the frequency of the dressing and tubing change. The SPS[22] recommends changing IV fluids tubing every 96 hours, transparent dressings every 7 days, and gauze dressings every 2 days, unless the integrity is compromised, and then it must be done sooner. Before a central line entry, SPS[22] recommends hand hygiene followed by disinfecting the hub or adapter with a friction scrub time of 15 seconds and allowing it to dry. Sterile gloves should be used anytime the hub is exposed (tubing and adapter changes) or when accessing a port with a needle.[22] Anyone in close proximity of the patient should wear a mask during a dressing change.[22] Using sterile gloves, clean the skin with friction using CHG for 30 seconds.[22] If the access site is femoral, then cleanse the site for 2 minutes and allow for complete drying.[22] Central line maintenance bundles can be complex and time consuming but are key to preventing CLABSI.

Maintenance bundles are most successful when nurses are provided with the assistive support and adequate time. In a single-center cross-sectional study from 160 surveys completed by bedside PICU nurses, greater than 90% recognized the importance of CLABSI bundles to families and hospital leadership.[24] One-third of the respondents reported forgetting a bundle component in the last 6 months.[24] Greater than 75% of the surveys reported meeting bundle requirements added stress to their shift and that their patient's care demands prevented them from meeting bundle compliance.[24] Other patient care tasks were delayed or prevented due to CLABSI bundle adherence, according to half of the surveys.[24] Woods-Hill and colleagues[24] found that the CLABSI bundle is the most time consuming but has greatest compliance when the PICU has a lower acuity and/or census and are provided with adequate support. High motivation to meet bundle compliance corresponded with high motivation by the provider team. Although a small sample size, there is evidence that patient care demands, assisting staff, and bundle education are challenges to meet bundle compliance.[24] Morris and colleagues[25] reported a decrease in CLABSI rates by 19% at Children's Hospital of Philadelphia by providing maintenance bundle education with a hands-on approach to both nurses and physicians. Education included dressing changes, adapter changes, line entries, and nursing empowerment for advocacy. Placement of central line adapter and tubing should avoid residing near areas of contamination such as the diaper area, gastric tube, and endotracheal tube or tracheostomy. Parents and nurses should perform tasks in order of clean to dirty, for example, accessing the central line or moving tubing connected to a central line before giving a medication through a gastric tube or performing diaper changes.[26] Thoughtful education and collaboration with the patient and family on caring for the central line and dressing will decrease the occurrence for unplanned dressing changes and contamination of the line (**Box 2**).

COVID-19

The novel coronavirus (SARS-CoV-2) responsible for the COVID-19 pandemic changed infection prevention practices in the health care system. Hand sanitizer utilization at one facility was increased by 4 times in a 2-month period.[27] Before the pandemic, hand hygiene compliance by health care workers when being visibly observed was 80% to 95%, in comparison to when being covertly observed, which was 30% to 50%.[27] Health care workers involved in direct and indirect care showed compliance consistently greater than 90% when COVID-19 erupted.[27] HAIs reduced significantly during the time of increased hand hygiene compliance, although there was a decrease in number of patient admissions, and this facility did not specifically

---

Box 2
Including patients and parents on maintenance bundles

Daily Rounds Participation
- Necessity
- Functionality
- Location
- Contamination
- Frequency of line entries
- Frequency of tubing changes (TPN, propofol, and so forth)
- Frequency of unplanned dressing changes

Dressing/Tubing Assessments
- Notify RN if nonocclusive or soiled
- Minimal touching of tubing/dressing
- Care that tubing rests least contaminated area

Aseptic Technique Collaboration
- Moments of hand hygiene (visitors and HCW)
- Everyone wear a mask when hub is exposed
- Scrub hub for 15 seconds before entry

Disinfecting
- Clean RN approved high touch surface areas (including cords attached to patient) q shift and if visibly soiled
- Designate a dirty diaper basin
- Daily linen/gown changes
- Daily CHG baths (>2 months of age)

Abbreviations: HCW, health care worker; RN, registered nurse; TPN, total parenteral nutrition.

Data from Children's Hospitals Solutions for Patient Safety. 2021. SPS prevention bundles. https://www.solutionsforpatientsafety.org/wp-content/uploads/SPS-Prevention-Bundles_FEB-2021.pdf

state the decrease in CLABSI. During the time of this study, hospitals experienced a shift in the number of people in the building to conserve patient protective equipment. Consults were deferred to a later date or provided remotely when possible, visitors were limited to only parents, and patient-to-nurse staffing ratios changed for those in isolation rooms.

SUMMARY

Although essential in the treatment of many PICU patients, central lines are the leading cause of infection in the PICU,[4] contributing to the morbidity and mortality of patients and increasing costs and length of stay.[2] PICU nurses play a key role in decreasing CLABSIs by adhering to strict hand hygiene[16] and using maintenance bundles.[24] Parents and families can be taught proper hand hygiene, allowing them to participate in their child's recovery by following infection control practices that can decrease the potential for a central line infection. By promoting a positive safety culture where a commitment to safety concerns is encouraged, nurses can contribute to successful infection control and decrease the CLABSI rate in the PICU.[21]

CLINICS CARE POINTS

- Educate patients and families on proper care for a central line and the importance in reducing infection.
- Educate patients and families on pathogen sources and vehicles.
- Promote a positive safety culture that enables communication amongst the team, including the patient and their family.

DISCLOSURE

The authors do not have any conflicts of interest or funding sources in the writing of this article.

REFERENCE

1. Hsu HE, Mathew R, Wang R, et al. Health care-associated infections among critically ill children in the US, 2013-2018. JAMA Pediatr 2020;e203223. https://doi.org/10.1001/jamapediatrics.2020.3223.
2. Goudie A, Dynan L, Brady PW, et al. Attributable cost and length of stay for central line-associated bloodstream infections. Pediatrics 2014;133(6):e1525-32.
3. Rosenthal VD, Al-Abdely HM, El-Kholy AA, et al. International nosocomial infection control consortium report, data summary of 50 countries for 2010-2015: Device-associated module. Am J Infect Control 2016;44(12):1495-504.
4. Martinez T, Baugnon T, Vergnaud E, et al. Central-line-associated bloodstream infections in a surgical paediatric intensive care unit: risk factors and prevention with chlorhexidine bathing. J Paediatr Child Health 2020;56(6):936-42.
5. Umscheid CA, Mitchell MD, Doshi JA, et al. Estimating the proportion of healthcare-associated infections that are reasonably preventable and the related mortality and costs. Infect Control Hosp Epidemiol 2011;32(2):101-14.
6. Gandra SI, Ellison RT 3rd. Modern trends in infection control practices in intensive care units. J Intensive Care Med 2014;29:311-26.

7. Best M, Neuhauser D. Ignaz Semmelweis and the birth of infection control. Qual Saf Health Care 2004;13(3):233–4.
8. McEnroe N. Celebrating florence Nightingale's bicentenary. Lancet 2020; 395(10235):1475–8.
9. Reef C. Florence nightingale: the courageous life of the legendary nurse. Boston, MA: Clarion Books; 2017.
10. Centers for Disease Control and Prevention. National healthcare and safety network (NHSN): bloodstream infection event (central-line associated bloodstream infection and non-central line associated bloodstream infection). 2021. Available at: https://www.cdc.gov/nhsn/pdfs/pscmanual/4psc_clabscurrent.pdf. Accessed March 30, 2021.
11. The Joint Commission. Preventing central line–associated bloodstream infections: useful tools, an international perspective. 2013. Available at: http://www. jointcommission.org/CLABSIToolkit. Accessed March 30, 2021.
12. Kleidon T, Ullman A. Right device assessment and selection in pediatrics. *Vessel Health and Preservation: The Right Approach for Vascular Access.* Springer; 2019. Available at: https://doi.org/10.1007/978-3-030-03149-7_14. Accessed August 30, 2021.
13. Patel N, Petersen TL, Simpson PM, et al. Rates of venous thromboembolism and central line-associated bloodstream infections among types of central venous access devices in critically ill children. Crit Care Med 2020;48(9):1340–8.
14. Badheka A, Bloxham J, Schmitz A, et al. Outcomes associated with peripherally inserted central catheters in hospitalised children: a retrospective 7-year single-centre experience. BMJ Open 2019;9(8). https://doi.org/10.1136/bmjopen-2018-026031. Available at: https://bmjopen.bmj.com/content/9/8/e026031.full.pdf.
15. Lake JG, Weiner LM, Milstone AM, et al. Pathogen distribution and antimicrobial resistance among pediatric healthcare-associated infections reported to the National healthcare safety network, 2011–2014. Infect Control Hosp Epidemiol 2018; 39(1):1–11. Available at: https://www.ncbi.nlm.nih.gov/pmc/articles/ PMC6643994/.
16. World Health Organization & WHO Patient Safety. WHO guidelines on hand hygiene in health care. 2009. Available at: https://www.who.int/publications/i/item/ 9789241597906. Accessed March 30, 2021.
17. Centers for Disease Control and Prevention. Central line-associated bloodstream infections: resources for patients and healthcare providers. 2011. Available at: https://www.cdc.gov/csels/dsepd/ss1978/lesson1/section10.html.   Accessed March 30, 2021.
18. The Joint Commission. National patient safety goals effective January 2021 for the   nursing   care   center   program.   2020.   Available   at: https://www. jointcommission.org/-/media/tjc/documents/standards/national-patient-safety-goals/2021/ncc_npsg_jan2021.pdf. Accessed March 30, 2021.
19. Campbell JI, Pham TT, Le T, et al. Facilitators and barriers to a family empowerment strategy to improve healthcare worker hand hygiene in a resource-limited setting. Am J Infect Control 2020;48(12):1485–90. Available at: https://www. ncbi.nlm.nih.gov/pubmed/32492500.
20. Arbogast JW, Moore L, Clark T, et al. Who goes in and out of patient rooms? An observational study of room entries and exits in the acute care setting. Am J Infect Control 2019;47(5):585–7. Available at: https://www.ncbi.nlm.nih.gov/ pubmed/30528169.
21. Braun BI, Chitavi SO, Suzuki H, et al. Culture of safety: impact on improvement in infection prevention process and outcomes. Curr Infect Dis Rep 2020;22(12).

https://doi.org/10.1007/s11908-020-00741-y. Available at: https://www.ncbi.nlm.nih.gov/pmc/articles/PMC7710367/.

22. Children's Hospitals Solutions for Patient Safety. SPS prevention bundles 2021. Available at: https://www.solutionsforpatientsafety.org/wp-content/uploads/SPS-Prevention-Bundles_FEB-2021.pdf.

23. Miller MR, Griswold M, Harris JM, et al. Decreasing PICU catheter-associated bloodstream infections: NACHRI's Quality Transformation efforts. Pediatrics 2010;125(2):206–13. Available at: https://www.ncbi.nlm.nih.gov/pubmed/20064860.

24. Woods-Hill CZ, Papili K, Nelson E, et al. Harnessing implementation science to optimize harm prevention in critically ill children: a pilot study of bedside nurse CLABSI bundle performance in the pediatric intensive care unit. Am J Infect Control 2020;49(3):345–51. Available at: https://www.ncbi.nlm.nih.gov/pubmed/32818579.

25. Morris K, Nelson E, Woods-Hill C. 1385 - PICU CLABSI Stand-Down education Back to basics. Crit Care Med 2019;47:669.

26. Joseph Y Ting, Vicki SK Goh Horacio Osiovich. Reduction of central line-associated bloodstream infection rates in a neonatal intensive care Unit after implementation of a Multidisciplinary evidence-based Quality improvement collaborative: a four-year Surveillance. Can J Infect Dis Med Microbiol 2013;24(4):185–90. Available at: https://www.ncbi.nlm.nih.gov/pubmed/24489559.

27. Stifter J, Sermersheim E, Ellsworth M, et al. COVID-19 and nurse-sensitive indicators - using performance improvement Teams to address Quality Indicators during a pandemic. J Nurs Care Qual 2021;36(1):1–6.

28. Centers for Disease Control and Prevention. Staphylococcus aureus in healthcare settings. 2011. Available at: https://www.cdc.gov/hai/organisms/staph.html. Accessed April 7, 2021.

29. Bush LM, Vazquez-Pertejo MT. Enterococcal infections. 2021. Available at: https://www.merckmanuals.com/professional/infectious-diseases/gram-positive-cocci/enterococcal-infections?query=enterococcus%20species. Accessed April 7, 2021.

30. Becker K, Heilmann C, Peters G. Coagulase-negative staphylococci. Clin Microbiol Rev 2014;27(4):870–926.

31. Ramirez D, Giron M. Enterobacter infections. Stat Pearls. 2021. Available at: https://www.ncbi.nlm.nih.gov/books/NBK559296/. Accessed April 7, 2021.

32. Centers for Disease Control and Prevention. Klebsiella pneumoniae in healthcare settings. 2010. Available at: https://www.cdc.gov/csels/dsepd/ss1978/lesson1/section10.html. Accessed April 7, 2021.

33. Centers for Disease Control and Prevention. Candidiasis. 2020. Available at: https://www.cdc.gov/fungal/diseases/candidiasis/index.html. Accessed April 7, 2021.

34. Centers for Disease Control and Prevention. Pseudomonas aeruginosa in healthcare settings. 2019. Available at: https://www.cdc.gov/hai/organisms/pseudomonas.html. Accessed April 7, 2021.

Special Articles

Evidence-Based Communication with Critically Ill Older Adults

JiYeon Choi, PhD, RN[a], Judith A. Tate, PhD, RN[b],*

KEYWORDS

- Communication • Mechanical ventilation
- Augmentative and alternative communication • Communication disorders
- Patient-centered care • Patient participation • Older adults

KEY POINTS

- Mechanical ventilation prohibits speech in critically ill patients.
- Being unable to communicate is frightening, frustrating and stressful for critically ill patients.
- Evidence-based methods to assess communication ability and select strategies to improve patient-clinician communication are important components of patient-centered care.

NATURE OF THE PROBLEM

Effective communication is the foundation of patient-centered care. Effective communication occurs when both the sender and receiver of messages achieve shared meaning and understanding.[1] Patient-centered communication builds on effective communication and includes patient perspectives, preferences, and choices. Furthermore, the patient's social and psychological context is valued as shared decision-making unfolds.[2]

The value of effective communication between health care providers and patients is acknowledged in health care accreditation standards as both a quality metric and as a fundamental patient right.[3] Communication failure is a critical factor in medical errors and in patient safety incidents.[4,5] Patients with communication impairments are at threefold risk for adverse events.[4] Despite the importance of communication to

This article originally appeared in The Critical Care Clinics, Volume 37, Issue 1, september 2020.
[a] Yonsei University College of Nursing, Mo-Im Kim Nursing Research Institute, 50-1 Yonsei-Ro, Seodaemun-Gu, Seoul 03722, Korea; [b] Center of Healthy Aging, Self-Management and Complex Care, Undergraduate Nursing Honors Program, The Ohio State University College of Nursing, 386 Newton Hall, 1585 Neil Avenue, Columbus, OH 43210, USA
* Corresponding author.
E-mail address: tate.230@osu.edu

improve patient care and outcomes, health care providers receive little or no training in evidence-based approaches in communication assessment and accommodation.[6]

In addition to preexisting communication disorders, patients may acquire communication impairments because of therapeutic interventions, such as mechanical ventilation, sedation, and neuromuscular blockade during critical illness. Endotracheal intubation or tracheostomy prevents patients' ability to vocalize, which is frightening, frustrating, and stressful.[7,8] Communication difficulty is one of the most common and most bothersome symptoms reported by patients undergoing mechanical ventilation (MV).[7,9–13] The inability to speak limits accurate identification of symptoms and can restrict participation in treatment decision-making.[7,8,11,12,14–16] The inability to communicate contributes to physical and emotional distress and predicts psychological distress in the post–intensive care unit (ICU) period.[17,18] Despite known communication difficulties in critically ill patients, interventions to support nonvocal patients with critical illness are poorly and inconsistently applied.[13,19,20]

Older adults, defined as older than 65 years, comprise approximately 50% of ICU admissions annually and as the aging population increases, this percentage is expected to grow.[21] Critically ill older adults present communication challenges based on their unique vulnerabilities such as burden of underlying chronic conditions, sensory impairment, frailty, and cognitive dysfunction[22–26] Most ICU health care providers learn how to communicate with impaired patients by trial and error or by observing others.[6]

This article presents an overview of evidence-based strategies to improve communication during the critical illness with older adults who have preexisting and acquired communication disorders due to hearing loss, vision impairment, limited English proficiency, health literacy, cognition, and limited upper extremity mobility.

Epidemiology of Preexisting Communication Disorders

- One in 6 people in the United States have a communication disorder.[27]
- Of these, 28 million have communication disorders associated with hearing loss.[28]
- 14 million people have disorders of speech, voice, and/or language not associated with hearing loss.[29]
- 90% of adults older than 50 require corrective lenses[30]
- 1 in 3 adults older than 65 has a hearing loss[24]

Communication disorders often occur concomitantly with other chronic disorders, such as diabetes, heart failure, stroke, renal disease, and dementia, contributing to a decreased ability to engage in self-management and resulting in high rates of disability.[30–35]

Hearing loss

Hearing loss is a common but underrecognized and undertreated problem in older adults.[36,37] Few studies provide direction for improving communication with patients who have hearing impairment.[33,38] Even with mild hearing loss, low levels of ambient noise competes with one-on-one communication.[38] Higher than normal noise levels in the ICU compound the effects of hearing loss.[39] During hospitalization, hearing aids are often removed and sent home because of their cost, which worsens communication and limits patient engagement.[25,40] Preexisting hearing impairment is associated with delirium and poor recovery following an ICU stay.[41,42] The use of hearing aids in the ICU both reduces the incidence of delirium and facilitates mobility.[43]

Health care professionals are often unaware of patients' hearing impairment and routine screening for hearing loss at the bedside lacks sensitivity.[26] Clinicians report difficulty communicating with patients with hearing loss, yet few receive formal training to develop skills necessary to resolve communication barriers.[38,44] Hearing loss is not always documented in the medical record and furthermore, few health care professionals are aware of how to access services for patients with hearing loss.[44]

A hearing assessment is necessary for all older patients admitted to the ICU. Evidence of hearing loss may be subtle and overlap with signs of other problems such as delirium. For instance, patients with hearing loss may not respond to verbal stimulus, which may be confused with inattention. Patients with hearing loss may be more responsive when they can see the communication partner's face. Clinicians may compound communication problems by rapid speech and/or use of medical jargon.[38]

An audiologist should evaluate patients with suspected or diagnosed preexisting hearing loss and can recommend simple strategies to accommodate patients with uncorrected hearing loss. Audiologists can troubleshoot problems with hearing aids and can provide brief bedside instructions to staff for appropriate use and care of hearing aids. In addition, audiologists can provide temporary hearing amplification devices if patients' own hearing aids are not available or if the hearing loss is uncorrected by hearing aids. Hearing aids should be available and inserted during the day to facilitate comprehension.[38,43,44]

Vision impairment

Given the high rates of visual impairment in all age groups and the increased prevalence of vision problems with aging, many patients require corrective lenses for reading or for distance vision correction. In older adults, visual impairment is associated with ICU delirium and poor recovery outcomes.[41] During hospitalization, patients are often expected to review educational materials, consent forms, and personal messages. Despite this, corrective lenses are not frequently made available for patients in the ICU.[45] Corrective lenses provide patients a way to make sense of their environment, identify caregivers, and compensate for hearing loss using lip-reading.

Limited English proficiency

Older adults in whom English is not their primary language may experience language barriers, making communication as well as comprehending medical terminology more difficult. Currently 1 in 15 adults are identified as Limited English Proficient (LEP) and with projected increases in immigration, this number is expected to increase.[46–48] Fifteen million older adults are LEP resulting in poor health and disparate health care access.[48,49] For any patients who are LEP, language access such as interpreter services and written materials in patients' native language are mandated now by the Affordable Care Act.

Cognitive impairment

Many patients with critical illness experience changes in their level of consciousness. Changes in cognitive function or delirium can result in changes in communication initiation and symptom communication.[16] Use of a standardized assessment tool such as the Confusion Assessment Method - ICU or Intensive Care Delirium Screening Checklist provide important data about the presence of delirium, acute confusion experienced by many ICU patients and common in older adults.[50,51] provide. Features common to delirium that may influence patient communication are impaired sustained attention, distorted thinking, inability to follow verbal commands, and changes in level of consciousness.[50,51]

Communicating with older adults may be further complicated by preexisting cognitive impairment. Impaired attention and focus are hallmark features of both delirium and dementia. Patients with delirium superimposed on dementia may have unpredictable communication patterns.[52] For instance, patients with dementia may have verbal fluency difficulties that the patient with delirium may not exhibit. Patients with dementia have slower cognitive processing speed making it difficult to understand and react to verbal input. Patients receiving sedating medications may also exhibit slower cognitive processing speed.

Because many patients experience delirium during their ICU stay, communication strategies directed at key features of delirium are imperative. To compensate for inattention, the clinician should initiate attention by facing the patient, establishing eye contact, and maintaining the face-to-face position.[53,54] Locking eyes can provide useful information for both the speaker and the patient.[53] The speaker can monitor patient engagement while the patient can see the speaker's mouth movement. Delays in comprehension may be due to cognitive impairment, sedation, fatigue, neurologic deficits, or hearing impairment.[55] Slowing the clinician's pace of speech and limiting ideas to one at a time can help to overcome delays in processing.[56] Increasing the duration of pauses between the sent message and the patient's response will allow the patient time to formulate a response. This technique can be useful in cases in which patients have motor slowing, as seen in Parkinson disease. Asking patients to confirm the sender's message or repeat the message may increase message accuracy and retention.[56]

Limited upper motor ability

ICU-acquired weakness (ICUAW) is profound neuromuscular dysfunction associated with critical illness and its treatment.[57,58] Preexisting functional impairment or frailty, common in older adults, is a risk factor for development of ICUAW.[57] Prolonged mechanical ventilation, sedation, and immobility are common and increase risk for ICUAW.[58] Patients with ICUAW exhibit decreased strength, muscle atrophy and decreased muscle mass, fatigue, weakness, and poor grip strength.[59] Effective communication strategies are limited by ICUAW. For instance, to write a message, patients should be able to sit upright, holding their head up, grip the pen, and produce a legible written message, ICUAW may prohibit use of writing as a strategy.

Pointing or gesturing is a common method of augmenting communication efforts and is an essential component for use of many communication strategies. If the patient can point, supportive communication strategies such as alphabet boards, picture boards or touch screens may be appropriate. Unfortunately, patients with critical illness may experience upper extremity edema, which can impair the ability to point or gesture. Use of sedating medications or paralytics will prevent use of pointing and writing. In addition, vascular access may make it difficult to move their extremities.[60,61]

Augmentative and Alternative Communication Strategies

Augmentative and alternative communication (AAC) strategies are a set of tools, technologies, and approaches used to overcome communication challenges that can be used to improve communication for voiceless patients in the ICU.[62] AAC strategies were originally developed to assist patients with acquired neurologic problems to communicate deficits but have been adapted by communication scientists to meet the needs of critically ill patients.[63] AAC strategies include unaided strategies (gestures, facial expressions, mouthing words), low-tech strategies (writing, letter boards) and high-tech strategies (computer-assisted devices, apps, speech-generating devices), as seen in **Table 1**.[19,63]

Adoption of AAC strategies in the ICU can lead to improved patient satisfaction with communication.[6,64,65] There are a variety of evidence-based methods to facilitate the

Table 1
Augmentative and alternative communication strategy classifications

Unaided *Nonspoken, natural*	Aided *Require external support*
Gestures Facial expression Body language Sign language	Communication boards Handheld devices Electronic devices

Low-tech strategies
  Strategy that does not
    require battery operated
    or electronic device
	High-tech strategies
	  Require energy source, electronic

Writing Picture boards Letter boards	Speech-generating devices Communication Apps VidaTalk LiveVoice Speak for Myself ICUTalk

use of AAC, including access to communication materials, and improving clinician knowledge and skills.[6,19,66–68] Barriers to use of AAC in the ICU include competing priorities for clinicians, as using AAC takes time away from other clinical activities.[6,67–69] Many clinicians limit communication exchanges with patients, as they have experienced frustration with communication breakdowns with nonspeaking patients.[70]

Low-tech strategies
Low-tech AAC include methods that enhance communication efforts using strategies and tools that do not require battery-operated devices. Communication boards include symbols, letters, pictures, icons, or a combination to facilitate messages by pointing by the patient or the clinician, as seen in **Fig. 1**. Communication boards can increase communication effectiveness and speed, decrease frustration, and improve patient satisfaction in communication with clinicians.[71,72] Communication boards, although the most restrictive option, are inexpensive, downloadable, and can be constructed on paper or purchased.

High-tech strategies
High-tech strategies include devices that use an electronic interface, as seen in **Fig. 2**.[64,73,74] Although more costly than low-tech strategies, some high-tech devices are able to generate speech in response to patients touching letters or symbols on the screen.[64,73–75] Some high-tech AACs use an application downloaded onto an electronic tablet.[76] Using the lettering feature enables patients to spell messages. To optimize effectiveness, patients should be alert and cognitively intact, unrestrained, and have the muscle strength and ability to point to icons.

Voice-enabling strategies
Several methods have been tested to enable speech generation by patients on MV. In their review of communication strategies for critically ill patients, Ten Hoorn and colleagues constructed an algorithm of voice-enabling strategies to guide clinical decision making when considering individualized communication interventions.[77]

The talking trach was designed to enable patients to generate vocal tones in a whisper, as seen in **Fig. 3**.[78] The cuff on the talking trach remains inflated, enabling

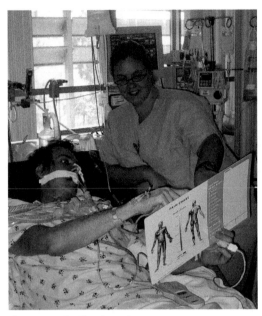

Fig. 1. Using low-tech communication board.

ventilation and vocalization as separate and safe functions. A talking trach tube necessitates a change in tube conferring a degree of risk of an airway exchange. Issues with secretion management with this device also make it a less desirable method.[78,79]

An inline speaking valve is a one-way airflow valve to enable vocalization. Use of an inline speaking valve requires deflation of the tracheostomy tube or the presence of a cuffless tracheostomy. The Passy-Muir valve improves vocal communication and cough, as illustrated in **Fig. 4**.[79] Use of the Passy-Muir valve is precluded in patients

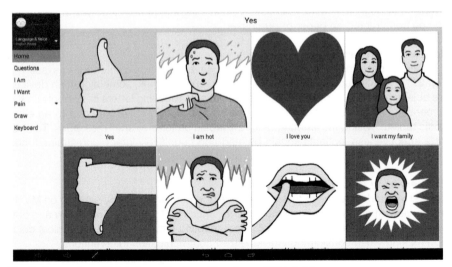

Fig. 2. Screen from Vidatalk application. (Courtesy of Vidatalk)

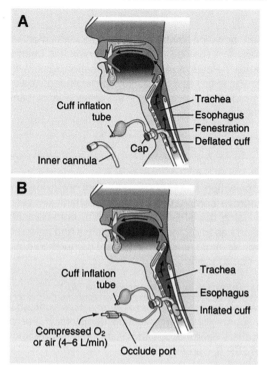

Fig. 3. (*A, B*) Talking Trach. (*A*) Fenestrated tracheostomy tube with cuff deflated, inner cannula removed, and tracheostomy tube capped to allow air to pass over the vocal cords. (*B*) Speaking tracheostomy tube. One tube is used for cuff inflation. (*From* Mathers, DM. Nursing Management. In: Heitkemper MM, Bucher Lin, Lewis SL, et al. (eds) Medical-Surgical Nursing: Assessment and Management of Clinical Problems, Ninth Edition, Philadelphia: Elsevier, 2014; with permission.)

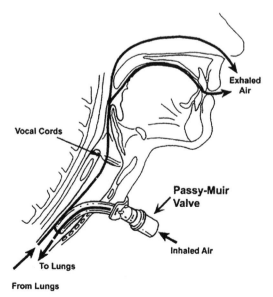

Fig. 4. Passy-Muir valve. (*From* Hodder RV. A 55-year-old patient with advanced COPD, tracheostomy tube, and sudden respiratory distress. Chest. 2002;121(1):279-280. https://doi.org/10.1378/chest.121.1.279; with permission.)

with heavy secretions, agitation, inability to maintain ventilation with a deflated cuff, and medical instability.[79,80] The use of an electrolarynx has been tested in mechanically ventilated patients.[81] Patients rated communication easier with the electrolarynx but its effectiveness was less when the patient experienced weakness.[81] In addition, patients required support for positioning the device and sentence intelligibility remained suboptimal.[81]

Communication Decision Support

Critically ill patients and their providers can learn to use communication aids in a systematic manner.[65,66] The SPEACS-2 algorithm is an evidence-based tool that guides patient assessment, selection of appropriate interventions to improve comprehension, and strategies to improve communication with mechanically ventilated patients, as seen in **Fig. 5**.[67,68] Using the SPEACS-2 algorithm, communication strategies can be attempted and used based on the patient's abilities and preferences. Communication strategies are not absolute, and as the patient's condition changes, communication approaches can be modified.

Speech Language Pathologists in the Intensive Care Unit

Speech language pathologists (SLPs) are experts in communication science and can be an invaluable resource for communication decisions.[82] For patients with more complex communication needs, such as those with neurologic disorders, expert consultation with an SLP is warranted.

Family Communication

Families often provide support and advocacy when patients are unable to speak for themselves.[83] Families experience distress when they are unable to communicate with the patient.[10,84,85] Patients on MV often appreciate the efforts of close relatives to understand them while they were unable to speak and families are likewise often interested in learning how to improve communication.[84,86] Studies have neither rigorously described patient-family communication in the ICU nor systematically tested communication strategies targeting families of the critically ill.

Engaging family members using telehealth

In the ICU setting, effectively engaging family members is essential. Information shared from family members is necessary to integrate data on a patient's medical, psychosocial, and behavioral history relevant to current illness. Support from family members can be represented a variety of ways, from providing silent companionship to actively responding and supporting patients' emotional and social needs.[86] Family members can be both surrogates and advocates, especially when the patient's communication ability is limited.[10,83,87,88] Efforts have been made to increase family presence in the ICU settings, such as using extended or open vitiation hours and inviting family to participate in daily ICU rounds.[89,90] However, family presence in the ICU is not always feasible. Decades of efforts to increase family presence in the ICU face a major barrier with the coronavirus 2019 (COVID-19) pandemic. Deprived access to family visits due to COVID-19 not only worsens suffering of patients and families but also adds stress to ICU clinicians.[91,92]

Telehealth, defined as the use of electronic information and telecommunication technologies to support health services delivery may be a timely solution to continue and improve family engagement for the critically ill.[93,94] In critical care, telehealth was initially introduced as a tool to reduce disparities in access to critical care workforces in rural areas.[95,96] Recently, family engagement has proven to be another area that

Low Tech Communication Strategies

STEP 1 – ASSESS

1. **COGNITION**
Is the patient alert?
Can they follow commands?
Can you raise your arm/make a fist?
Blink your eyes twice.

2. **ORAL MOTOR MOVEMENT**
Are the patient's mouth movements clear when
mouthing speech?
Count from 1 to 10.
Tell me about your first job in a sentence.

3. **COMPREHENSION**
Does the patient need help with comprehension?
Do they wear glasses/hearing aids?
Are they available?
Any language barriers?

4. **EXPRESSIVE COMMUNICATION**
Does the patient have a reliable yes/no signal?
How does the patient signal yes?
How does the patient signal no?

Can the patient point?
Can the patient write?

Assess language and literacy
Engage SLP or translation services if non-English
speaking or unable to read.

STEP II - PROVIDE COMPREHENSION STRATEGIES

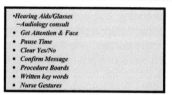

- *Hearing Aids/Glasses*
  - *–Audiology consult*
- *Get Attention & Face*
- *Pause Time*
- *Clear Yes/No*
- *Confirm Message*
- *Procedure Boards*
- *Written key words*
- *Nurse Gestures*

STEP III – CHOOSE STRATEGY BASED ON ORAL MOTOR SKILL

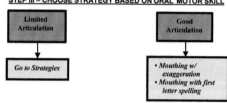

STEP IV – CHOOSE STRATEGIES FOR EXPRESSIVE COMMUNICATION

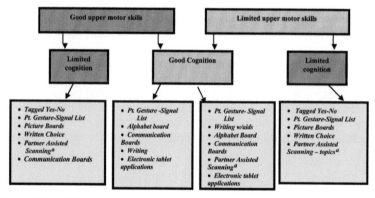

Fig. 5. SPEACS-2 algorithm.[a] Consult speech language pathologist (SLP) for complex strategies or if selected strategies are unsuccessful. (©Garret, Happ, Tate 2006 (Revised 2009: SPEACS-2; 2016) R01 HD043988.)

may benefit from telehealth. Telehealth is a solution to help family members maintain connections with patients and participate in both communication and decision making with the health care team.

A simple approach, for example, playing the audio-recorded voice of family members, can benefit both patients and families. Munro and colleagues[97] developed and pilot-tested a cognitive reorientation intervention to prevent delirium in critically ill patients. In their intervention, family members were instructed to read and record a scripted 2-minute message and the recorded message was played in the patient's room. Reorientation messages include orientation of the patient's current location and reasons for physical limitations (eg, endotracheal tube). Results of this randomized controlled trial demonstrated preliminary efficacy in reducing delirium.

Video-conferencing and Web-based portals may be the most popular technologies considered for family engagement. Video-conferencing sets up real-time interactions between 2 or more parties, whereas Web-based portals may have conferencing capabilities but also have pre-posted information or patient centered apps, for example, VidaTalk. Various commercial online platforms are now Health Insurance Portability and Accountability Act (HIPAA)-compliant. Despite their potential to promote family engagement, establishing evidence specific to gero-critical care settings is a remaining step for its real-world application. For example, video-conferencing technologies may appear to be an obvious solution to promote real-time engagement of family members in patient visits, ICU clinical team rounds, and family meetings.[98–102] However, the acceptance by families or clinicians of the use of video conferencing for virtual family rounds, varies.[103] Most family members and clinicians are supportive of the idea of virtual rounds; however, family members have varying levels of technology literacy and comfort levels. Some clinicians expressed concerns of adding burden to their clinical workload.[103]

Another example of using telehealth to engage family members includes interactive online decision-support programs to guide complex surrogate decision making, such as goals of treatment.[104,105] Guided by theories addressing both cognitive and emotional aspects of decision making, online decision-support programs have made rapid developments.[104] Although the initial program was mainly based on the cognitive aspects of surrogate decision making, a recent development added a tool to support the emotional and psychological challenges that families experience during decision making.[104,105] These programs were suggested as an adjunct to help families prepare for complex conversations during in-person meetings with the ICU clinical team.[105]

The aforementioned technologies, from the use of a voice recording device to communication and/or decision-aid software, highlight the different media available to improve family engagement in the ICU. In the process of adopting these technologies, attention should also be paid to disparities in access to the technology, digital literacy, and Internet access among the family members. Efforts to resolve these disparities are important to ensure people with fewer resources and access are included.

Box 1
Communication resources

Communication resources
  Patient-Provider Communication Organization
  https://www.patientprovidercommunication.org/

Communication training
  https://nucleus.con.ohio-state.edu/media/speacs2/project_desc.htm

Organizations
  US Society for Augmentative and Alternative Communication
  https://ussaac.org/
  International Society for Augmentative and Alternative Communication
  https://www.isaac-online.org/english/home/
  American Speech Language Hearing Association
  https://www.asha.org/

SUMMARY

Losing the ability to speak while on MV can be a frightening and frustrating experience for patients. Effective communication with mechanically ventilated patients is a critical component of patient-centered care. Given the number of older adults in the ICU with preexisting communication disorders and cognitive impairment, older adults are at greater risk for communication breakdown in the ICU. Communication assessment and selection of appropriate strategies should be approached systematically. Additional resources can be found in **Box 1**.

CLINICS CARE POINTS

Recommendations for ICU Practice Change Related to Communication
- *ICU rounds*: During ICU rounds, the clinicians should be able to answer: (1) Is the patient communicating effectively? If yes, using what mechanism? (2) Is a sign posted in the patient's room denoting communication difficulty? (3) Has a speech language pathologist been consulted? If so, what are their recommendations? and (4) Has there been a change in the patient's condition that might affect their communication ability?
- *Documentation*: Nurses should systematically and routinely chart the patient's communication function: (1) How are they communicating overall, and specifically their ability to communicate "yes" and "no"? and (2) Are there changes in patient's condition that might affect their communication ability?
- *Communication plans:* A communication plan should be posted by the patient's bed that lists how the patient is able to both (1) convey thoughts, needs, and symptoms accurately to their providers, and (2) understands what care providers are communicating, including sensory aids (eg, glasses, hearing aids).

DISCLOSURE

JiYeon Choi was supported by National Research Foundation (NRF) of Korea (2019R1F1A1057941). The other author have no conflicts to disclose.

REFERENCES

1. Fleischer S, Berg A, Zimmermann M, et al. Nurse-patient interaction and communication: a systematic literature review. J Public Health 2009;17(5): 339–53.
2. Slatore CG, Hansen L, Ganzini L, et al. Communication by nurses in the intensive care unit: qualitative analysis of domains of patient-centered care. Am J Crit Care 2012;21(6):410–8.
3. JCAHO. Patient-centered communication standards for hospitals. 2011.
4. Bartlett G, Blais R, Tamblyn R, et al. Impact of patient communication problems on the risk of preventable adverse events in acute care settings. CMAJ 2008; 178(12):1555–62.
5. Hemsley B, Georgiou A, Hill S, et al. An integrative review of patient safety in studies on the care and safety of patients with communication disabilities in hospital. Patient Educ Couns 2016;99(4):501–11.
6. Magnus VS, Turkington L. Communication interaction in icu—patient and staff experiences and perceptions. Intensive Crit Care Nurs 2006;22(3):167–80.

7. Rotondi AJ, Chelluri L, Sirio C, et al. Patients' recollections of stressful experiences while receiving prolonged mechanical ventilation in an intensive care unit. Crit Care Med 2002;30(4):746–52.

8. Guttormson JL, Bremer KL, Jones RM. "Not being able to talk was horrid": a descriptive, correlational study of communication during mechanical ventilation. Intensive Crit Care Nurs 2015;31(3):179–86.

9. Nelson JE, Meier DE, Litke A, et al. The symptom burden of chronic critical illness. Crit Care Med 2004;32(7):1527–34.

10. Happ MB. Interpretation of nonvocal behavior and the meaning of voicelessness in critical care. Social Sci Med 2000;50(9):1247–55.

11. Danielis M, Povoli A, Mattiussi E, et al. Understanding patients' experiences of being mechanically ventilated in the intensive care unit: Findings from a meta-synthesis and meta-summary. J Clin Nurs 2020;29(13–14):2107–24.

12. Fink RM, Makic MBF, Poteet AW, et al. The ventilated patient's experience. Dimensions Crit Care Nurs 2015;34(5):301–8.

13. Freeman-Sanderson A, Morris K, Elkins M. Characteristics of patient communication and prevalence of communication difficulty in the intensive care unit: an observational study. Aust Crit Care 2019;32(5):373–7.

14. Karlsen MMW, Ølnes MA, Heyn LG. Communication with patients in intensive care units: a scoping review. Nurs Crit Care 2019;24(3):115–31.

15. Tate JA, Seaman JB, Happ MB. Overcoming barriers to pain assessment: communicating pain information with intubated older adults. Geriatr Nurs (New York, NY). 2012;33(4):310–3.

16. Tate JA, Sereika S, Divirgilio D, et al. Symptom communication during critical illness: the impact of age, delirium, and delirium presentation. J Gerontol Nurs 2013;39(8):28–38.

17. Wade DM, Howell DC, Weinman JA, et al. Investigating risk factors for psychological morbidity three months after intensive care: a prospective cohort study. Crit Care 2012;16(5):R192.

18. Parker AM, Sricharoenchai T, Raparla S, et al. Posttraumatic stress disorder in critical illness survivors: a metaanalysis. Crit Care Med 2015;43(5):1121–9.

19. Istanboulian L, Rose L, Gorospe F, et al. Barriers to and facilitators for the use of augmentative and alternative communication and voice restorative strategies for adults with an advanced airway in the intensive care unit: a scoping review. J Crit Care 2020;57:168–76.

20. Hurtig RR, Downey D. Augmentative and alternative communication in acute and critical care settings. San Diego (CA): Plural Publishing; 2008.

21. Zilberberg MD, de Wit M, Shorr AF. Accuracy of previous estimates for adult prolonged acute mechanical ventilation volume in 2020: Update using 2000–2008 data. Crit Care Med 2012;40(1):18–20.

22. Ferrante LE, Pisani MA, Murphy TE, et al. The association of frailty with post-icu disability, nursing home admission, and mortality: a longitudinal study. Chest. 2018;153(6):1378–86.

23. He Z, Bian J, Carretta HJ, et al. Prevalence of multiple chronic conditions among older adults in Florida and the United States: Comparative analysis of the one-florida data trust and national inpatient sample. J Med Internet Res 2018;20(4): e137.

24. National Institute on Deafness and Other Communication Disorders. Hearing loss and older adults. 2016. Available at: https://www.nidcd.nih.gov/health/hearing-loss-older-adults.

25. Funk A, Garcia C, Mullen T. Ce: Original research understanding the hospital experience of older adults with hearing impairment. AJN The Am J Nurs 2018;118(6):28–34.

26. Mormer E, Bubb KJ, Alrawashdeh M, et al. Hearing loss and communication among hospitalized older adults: prevalence and recognition. J Gerontol Nurs 2020;46(6):34–42.

27. Healthy People.gov. Hearing and other sensory or communication disorders. 2014. Available at: https://www.healthypeople.gov/2020/topics-objectives/topic/hearing-and-other-sensory-or-communication-disorders. Accessed July 31, 2020.

28. Hoffman HJ, Dobie RA, Losonczy KG, et al. Declining prevalence of hearing loss in us adults aged 20 to 69 years. JAMA Otolaryngol Head Neck Surg 2017;143(3):274–85.

29. Blackwell DL, Lucas JW, Clarke TC. Summary health statistics for us adults: national health interview survey, 2012. Vital Health Stat Ser 10 2014;(260):1–161.

30. The National Eye Institute. Eye health data and statistics. 2019. Available at: https://www.nei.nih.gov/learn-about-eye-health/resources-for-health-educators/eye-health-data-and-statistics. Accessed July 31, 2020.

31. Flowers HL, Skoretz SA, Silver FL, et al. Poststroke aphasia frequency, recovery, and outcomes: a systematic review and meta-analysis. Arch Phys Med Rehabil 2016;97(12):2188–201.e8.

32. Froehlich-Grobe K, Jones D, Businelle MS, et al. Impact of disability and chronic conditions on health. Disabil Health J 2016;9(4):600–8.

33. Moore S. Scientific reasons for including persons with disabilities in clinical and translational diabetes research. J Diabetes Sci Tech 2012;6(2):236–41.

34. Nantsupawat A, Wichaikhum OA, Abhichartibutra K, et al. Nurses' knowledge of health literacy, communication techniques, and barriers to the implementation of health literacy programs: a cross-sectional study. Nurs Health Sci 2020;22(3):577–85.

35. Mirza M, Harrison EA, Roman M, et al. Walking the talk: understanding how language barriers affect the delivery of rehabilitation services. Disabil Rehabil 2020;1–14.

36. Goman AM, Reed NS, Lin FR. Addressing estimated hearing loss in adults in 2060. JAMA Otolaryngol Head Neck Surg 2017;143(7):733–4.

37. Lin FR, Niparko JK, Ferrucci L. Hearing loss prevalence in the United States. Arch Intern Med 2011;171(20):1851–3.

38. Cohen JM, Blustein J, Weinstein BE, et al. Studies of physician-patient communication with older patients: how often is hearing loss considered? A systematic literature review. J Am Geriatr Soc 2017;65(8):1642–9.

39. Konkani A, Oakley B. Noise in hospital intensive care units—a critical review of a critical topic. J Crit Care 2012;27(5):522.e1-9.

40. Hardin SR. Hearing loss in older critical care patients: participation in decision making. Crit Care Nurse 2012;32(6):43–50.

41. Ferrante LE, Pisani MA, Murphy TE, et al. Factors associated with functional recovery among older intensive care unit survivors. Am J Respir Crit Care Med 2016;194(3):299–307.

42. Inouye SK, Viscoli CM, Horwitz RI, et al. A predictive model for delirium in hospitalized elderly medical patients based on admission characteristics. Ann Intern Med 1993;119(6):474–81.

43. Vidán MT, Sánchez E, Alonso M, et al. An intervention integrated into daily clinical practice reduces the incidence of delirium during hospitalization in elderly patients. J Am Geriatr Soc 2009;57(11):2029–36.
44. Shukla A, Nieman CL, Price C, et al. Impact of hearing loss on patient–provider communication among hospitalized patients: a systematic review. Am J Med Qual 2019;34(3):284–92.
45. Zhou Q, Walker NF. Promoting vision and hearing aids use in an intensive care unit. BMJ Open Qual 2015;4(1). u206276.w2702.
46. Passel J, Rohal M. Modern immigration wave brings 59 million to US, driving population growth and change through 2065: Views of immigration's impact on US society mixed. Washington, DC: Pew Research Center; 2015. Available at: https://www.pewresearch.org/hispanic/wp-content/uploads/sites/5/2015/09/2015-09-28_modern-immigration-wave_REPORT.pdf.
47. US Census Bureau. Language use. 2019. Available at: https://www.census.gov/topics/population/language-use.html. Accessed September 18, 2020.
48. LEP.gov. Limited English proficiency (LEP) frequently asked questions. Available at: https://www.lep.gov/faqs/faqs.html#OneQ1. Accessed September 20, 2020.
49. Derose KP, Escarce JJ, Lurie N. Immigrants and health care: sources of vulnerability. Health Aff 2007;26(5):1258–68.
50. Devlin JW, Fong JJ, Schumaker G, et al. Use of a validated delirium assessment tool improves the ability of physicians to identify delirium in medical intensive care unit patients. Crit Care Med 2007;35(12):2721–4.
51. Ely EW, Margolin R, Francis J, et al. Evaluation of delirium in critically ill patients: validation of the confusion assessment method for the intensive care unit (CAM-ICU). Crit Care Med 2001;29(7):1370–9.
52. Fick DM, Agostini JV, Inouye SK. Delirium superimposed on dementia: a systematic review. J Am Geriatr Soc 2002;50(10):1723–32.
53. Frischen A, Bayliss AP, Tipper SP. Gaze cueing of attention: visual attention, social cognition, and individual differences. Psychol Bull 2007;133(4):694.
54. Poliakoff E, Ashworth S, Lowe C, et al. Vision and touch in ageing: Crossmodal selective attention and visuotactile spatial interactions. Neuropsychologia. 2006;44(4):507–17.
55. Savundranayagam MY, Orange JB. Matched and mismatched appraisals of the effectiveness of communication strategies by family caregivers of persons with alzheimer's disease. Int J Lang Commun Disord 2014;49(1):49–59.
56. Eccles DR. Communicating with the cognitively impaired patient. Florida Board of Nursing. Tallahassee (FL): Advance Nursing Institute INC; 2013.
57. Vanhorebeek I, Latronico N, Van den Berghe G. ICU-acquired weakness. Intensive Care Med 2020;150(5):1129–40.
58. Fan E, Cheek F, Chlan L, et al. An official American Thoracic Society clinical practice guideline: the diagnosis of intensive care unit–acquired weakness in adults. Am J Respir Crit Care Med 2014;190(12):1437–46.
59. Chlan LL, Tracy MF, Guttormson J, et al. Peripheral muscle strength and correlates of muscle weakness in patients receiving mechanical ventilation. Am J Crit Care 2015;24(6):e91–8.
60. Beukelman DR, Garrett KL, Yorkston KM. Augmentative communication strategies for adults with acute or chronic medical conditions. Baltimore (MD): Paul H. Brookes Publishing Company; 2007.
61. Happ MB, Seaman JB, Nilsen ML, et al. The number of mechanically ventilated ICU patients meeting communication criteria. Heart & Lung 2015;44(1):45-9.

62. International society for augmentative and alternative communication.What is AAC? 2014. Available at: https://www.isaac-online.org/english/what-is-aac/. Accessed July 31, 2020.

63. Carruthers H, Astin F, Munro W. Which alternative communication methods are effective for voiceless patients in intensive care units? A systematic review. Intensive Crit Care Nurs 2017;42:88–96.

64. Rodriguez CS, Rowe M, Koeppel B, et al. Development of a communication intervention to assist hospitalized suddenly speechless patients. Technology Health Care 2012;20(6):519–30.

65. Happ MB, Garrett KL, Tate JA, et al. Effect of a multi-level intervention on nurse-patient communication in the intensive care unit: results of the speacs trial. Heart Lung. 2014;43(2):89–98.

66. Happ MB, Sereika SM, Houze MP, et al. Quality of care and resource use among mechanically ventilated patients before and after an intervention to assist nurse-nonvocal patient communication. Heart & Lung. 2015;44(5):408–15.e2.

67. Trotta RL, Hermann RM, Polomano RC, et al. Improving nonvocal critical care patients' ease of communication using a modified speacs-2 program. J Healthc Qual (Jhq) 2020;42(1):e1–9.

68. Radtke JV, Tate JA, Happ MB. Nurses' perceptions of communication training in the icu. Intensive Crit Care Nurs 2012;28(1):16–25.

69. Dithole K, Thupayagale-Tshweneagae G, Akpor OA, et al. Communication skills intervention: promoting effective communication between nurses and mechanically ventilated patients. BMC Nurs 2017;16(1):74.

70. Holm A, Dreyer P. Use of communication tools for mechanically ventilated patients in the intensive care unit. CIN: Comput Inform Nurs 2018;36(8):398–405.

71. Otuzoğlu M, Karahan A. Determining the effectiveness of illustrated communication material for communication with intubated patients at an intensive care unit. Int J Nurs Pract 2014;20(5):490–8.

72. Patak L, Gawlinski A, Fung NI, et al. Communication boards in critical care: patients' views. Appl Nurs Res 2006;19(4):182–90.

73. Happ MB, Roesch TK, Garrett K. Electronic voice-output communication aids for temporarily nonspeaking patients in a medical intensive care unit: a feasibility study. Heart & Lung. 2004;33(2):92–101.

74. Koszalinski RS, Tappen RM, Viggiano D. Evaluation of speak for myself with patients who are voiceless. Rehabil Nurs J 2015;40(4):235–42.

75. Miglietta MA, Bochicchio G, Scalea TM. Computer-assisted communication for critically ill patients: a pilot study. J Trauma 2004;57(3):488–93.

76. Happ MB, Von Visger T, Weber ML, et al. Iterative development, usability, and acceptability testing of a communication app for mechanically ventilated patients. Am J Resp Crit Care Med 2016;193:A1096.

77. Ten Hoorn S, Elbers P, Girbes A, et al. Communicating with conscious and mechanically ventilated critically ill patients: a systematic review. Crit Care 2016;20(1):333.

78. Hess DR. Facilitating speech in the patient with a tracheostomy. Respir Care 2005;50(4):519–25.

79. Zaga CJ, Berney S, Vogel AP. The feasibility, utility, and safety of communication interventions with mechanically ventilated intensive care unit patients: a systematic review. Am J speech-language Pathol 2019;28(3):1335–55.

80. O'Connor LR, Morris NR, Paratz J. Physiological and clinical outcomes associated with use of one-way speaking valves on tracheostomised patients: a systematic review. Heart & Lung. 2019;48(4):356–64.

81. Rose L, Istanboulian L, Smith OM, et al. Feasibility of the electrolarynx for enabling communication in the chronically critically ill: the eeccho study. J Crit Care 2018;47:109–13.

82. Blackstone SW, Pressman H. Patient communication in health care settings: new opportunities for augmentative and alternative communication. Augment Altern Commun 2016;32(1):69–79.

83. Happ MB, Swigart VA, Tate JA, et al. Family presence and surveillance during weaning from prolonged mechanical ventilation. Heart & Lung. 2007;36(1):47–57.

84. Broyles LM, Tate JA, Happ MB. Use of augmentative and alternative communication strategies by family members in the intensive care unit. Am J Crit Care 2012;21(2):e21–32.

85. Alasad J, Ahmad M. Communication with critically ill patients. J Adv Nurs 2005;50(4):356–62.

86. Engstrom A, Soderberg S. The experiences of partners of critically ill persons in an intensive care unit. Intensive Crit Care Nurs 2004;20(5):299–308 [quiz: 309–210].

87. Scheunemann LP, Ernecoff NC, Buddadhumaruk P, et al. Clinician-family communication about patients' values and preferences in intensive care units. JAMA Intern Med 2019;179(5):676–84.

88. Shin JW, Tate JA, Happ MB. The facilitated sensemaking model as a framework for family-patient communication during mechanical ventilation in the intensive care unit. Crit Care Nurs Clin North Am 2020;32(2):335–48.

89. Liu V, Read JL, Scruth E, et al. Visitation policies and practices in us icus. Crit Care 2013;17(2):1–7.

90. Au SS, des Ordons ALR, Leigh JP, et al. A multicenter observational study of family participation in ICU rounds. Crit Care Med 2018;46(8):1255–62.

91. Kotfis K, Williams Roberson S, Wilson JE, et al. Covid-19: ICU delirium management during sars-cov-2 pandemic. Crit Care 2020;24:1–9.

92. Greenberg N, Docherty M, Gnanapragasam S, et al. Managing mental health challenges faced by healthcare workers during covid-19 pandemic. BMJ 2020;368.

93. HealthIT. gov. What is telehealth? How is telehealth different from telemedicine?. Available at: https://www.healthit.gov/faq/what-telehealth-how-telehealth-different-telemedicine. Accessed July 31, 2020.

94. Calton B, Abedini N, Fratkin M. Telemedicine in the time of coronavirus. J Pain Symptom Management. 2020;60(1):e12–4.

95. Lilly CM, Zubrow MT, Kempner KM, et al. Critical care telemedicine: evolution and state of the art. Crit Care Med 2014;42(11):2429–36.

96. Kahn JM, Cicero BD, Wallace DJ, et al. Adoption of intensive care unit telemedicine in the United States. Crit Care Med 2014;42(2):362.

97. Munro CL, Cairns P, Ji M, et al. Delirium prevention in critically ill adults through an automated reorientation intervention–a pilot randomized controlled trial. Heart & Lung. 2017;46(4):234–8.

98. Olanipekun T, Ezeagu R, Oni O, et al. Improving the quality of family participation in ICU rounds through effective communication and telemedicine. Read Online Crit Care Med Soy Cril Care Me 2019;47(2):e159.

99. Menon PR, Stapleton RD, McVeigh U, et al. Telemedicine as a tool to provide family conferences and palliative care consultations in critically ill patients at rural health care institutions: a pilot study. Am J Hosp Palliat Medicine®. 2015;32(4):448–53.

100. Østervang C, Vestergaard LV, Dieperink KB, et al. Patient rounds with video-consulted relatives: qualitative study on possibilities and barriers from the perspective of healthcare providers. J Med Internet Res 2019;21(3):e12584.
101. Yager PH, Clark M, Cummings BM, et al. Parent participation in pediatric intensive care unit rounds via telemedicine: feasibility and impact. J Pediatr 2017; 185:181-6.e3.
102. de Havenon A, Petersen C, Tanana M, et al. A pilot study of audiovisual family meetings in the intensive care unit. J Crit Care 2015;30(5):881-3.
103. Stelson EA, Carr BG, Golden KE, et al. Perceptions of family participation in intensive care unit rounds and telemedicine: a qualitative assessment. Am J Crit Care 2016;25(5):440-7.
104. Cox CE, White DB, Hough CL, et al. Effects of a personalized web-based decision aid for surrogate decision makers of patients with prolonged mechanical ventilation: a randomized clinical trial. Ann Intern Med 2019;170(5):285-97.
105. Suen AO, Butler RA, Arnold R, et al. Developing the family support tool: an interactive, web-based tool to help families navigate the complexities of surrogate decision making in icus. J Crit Care 2020;56:132-9.

TeleICU Interdisciplinary Care Teams

Cindy Welsh, RN, MBA[a],[1],*, Teresa Rincon, PhD, RN, CCRN-k[b],
Iris Berman, MSN, BSN, RN, CCRN-k[c], Tom Bobich, MBA[d],[2], Theresa Brindise, MS, BSN, RN[e],[1],
Theresa Davis, PhD, RN, NE-BC[f]

KEYWORDS

- Interdisciplinary • TeleICU • Staffing • Work flow • Remote ICU • TeleICU team
- Intensive care

KEY POINTS

- The composition of the TeleICU team requires several key factors to be evaluated; one size does not fit all.
- Workflows in the TeleICU are established by key stakeholders, including the bedside caregivers and the TeleICU team, while incorporating evidence-based best practices.
- TeleICU technology facilitates collaborative and integrated workflows.

INTRODUCTION

The terms telemedicine and telehealth are considered interchangeable terms by the American Telemedicine Association and are defined as the use of remote health care technologies to deliver health care services.[1] Telehealth in intensive care units (TeleICU) is the provision of critical care using audio-visual communication and health information systems to leverage expertise and decision support systems across varying clinical and geographically dispersed settings.[2],[3] TeleICU care includes 2 geographic components: the TeleICU care center (referred to as the "hub" or distant

This article originally appeared in The Critical Care Clinics, Volume 35, Issue 3, february 2019.
C. Welsh, I. Berman, T. Bobich, and T. Brindise have no commercial or financial conflicts to disclose. T. Rincon has received travel support (no honorarium) by Philips Healthcare for advisory and speaking roles. T. Davis is a Director on the AACN Board of Directors.
[a] Adult Critical Care, eICU, AdvocateAuroraHealth, 1400 Kensington Road, Oak Brook, IL 60523, USA; [b] Graduate School of Nursing, University of Massachusetts Medical School, 55 Lake Avenue North, Worcester, MA 01655, USA; [c] Telehealth Services, Northwell Health, 15 Burke Lane, Syosset, NY 11791, USA; [d] VP - Marketing, Hicuity Health, 2040 Main Street Suite 240, Irvine, CA 92614, USA; [e] AdvocateAuroraHealth, eICU, 1400 Kensington Road, Oak Brook, IL 60523, USA; [f] enVision TeleICU Inova Telemedicine, Inova Transfer Center, 8110 Gatehouse Road Suite 600 West, Falls Church, VA 22042, USA
[1] Present address: 1901 S. Meyers Road, Suite 410B, Oak Brook Terrace, IL 60181.
[2] Present address: 2040 Main Street, Suite 240, Irvine, CA 92614.
* Corresponding author. 1400 Kensington Road, Oak Brook, IL 60523.
E-mail address: cindy.welsh@aah.org

site) and the hospital critical care environment (referred to as the origin or spoke site) where the patient is receiving care from the hub with the support of the telemedicine technology.[1,4] This article focuses on the predominant TeleICU model, which uses continuous monitoring and a centralized hub (or multiple hubs). Some TeleICU models use an episodic consultative approach to intervention, whereby distant clinicians intervene remotely only when contacted by the site. The efficacy and cost of this model could be evaluated when considering the use of remote TeleICU.[5–8]

The technology platforms for telehealth include components of hardware, software, and mobile applications (apps) to optimize the surveillance and care of patients for the provider and receiver of services.[3] Information related to the optimal TeleICU team structure is lacking in the literature. This article examines the optimal TeleICU team composition, which is one that incorporates the use of an interdisciplinary approach, leverages technology, and is cognizant of varying geographic locations. In addition, the American Association of Critical Care Nurses (AACN) Synergy Model and Healthy Work Environments (HWE) standards, and the Relational Coordination theoretic foundation, are discussed. Use of these models is important to the development, composition, and success of the TeleICU team.[2,9] Finally, future possibilities for TeleICU team structures and functions are discussed as telemedicine continues to evolve and finds its way into mainstream medicine as an integral component of the health care system.

THE ESSENTIAL TeleICU TEAM STRUCTURE

The optimal structure of a TeleICU team is one that leverages expert clinical knowledge to address the needs of critical care patients, regardless of hospital geography or availability of an onsite intensivist. Early applications in 1999 focused on an intensivist-driven care model working in synergy with expert critical care nurses in the distant site.[10,11] Through the evolution of critical care, the importance of a team approach that combines the efforts of all team members, regardless of their physical location and inclusive of both origin and distant site locations, to achieve optimal care delivery in complex critical care environments has been revealed.[12] Failing to understand this cohesive view of a care team in a variety of settings risks a focus on the distant site that narrowly prescribes a solution certain to be deemed insufficient in today's health care environment. As the complexity of care increases for the critically ill patient, the necessity of a collaborative care team at the hub and spoke sites becomes more apparent.

TeleICU staffing models vary in the number of nurses and physicians to patients or beds. This variability depends on the workflow and support provided, resources available, and initiatives to control the cost of the TeleICU program.[3] Staffing structures should be established, and then evolve, based on the needs of the intensive care units (ICUs) that are supported by the TeleICU. These needs may differ among various ICUs and can be dynamic over shifts, suggesting that TeleICU staffing might look quite different overnight or over the weekend in comparison with a daytime shift.

According to Kahn and colleagues,[13] there are 4 major ways that TeleICU teams provide services: (1) monitor for physiologic deterioration, (2) diffusion of evidence-based practice, (3) expert advice and guidance, and (4) collecting, auditing, analyzing, and disseminating quality performance data. TeleICU staffing and workflows will differ based on the makeup of the bedside team. For example, in ICUs that lack intensivists on site, having around-the-clock presence of intensivists in the TeleICU to support evidence-based care decisions can improve patient outcomes. The TeleICU may augment intensivist and/or the advanced practice provider (APP) presence in the ICU to assist with managing multiple simultaneous demands or to provide support when the intensivist is not present. Intensivist presence in the TeleICU might not be around-the-clock; they may be present in higher-demand periods, and their workflows might call for them to advise and defer to the bedside team consistently. Technology capabilities and compatibilities and access to various software programs used in patient management will also impact team structure to a significant extent.

TeleICU TEAM MEMBERS

Most TeleICU clinical teams consist of a group of expert critical care nurses working with 1 or more physicians (generally intensivists) to support the care of critically ill and injured patients regardless of the patient's (and potentially the clinician's) location.[3,14,15] Some TeleICUs also use other disciplines, such as nurse practitioners, physician assistants, collectively referred to as APPs, as well as pharmacists and others.[3,14] Nonclinical support roles such as data assistant, clerical support, technical support, and quality and reporting analysts can round out the TeleICU team. Some of these variations will be discussed later in this article. Although this article will focus on clinical roles, the nonclinical positions are key to optimizing the role of the clinicians and their ability to function at the top of their license by providing clerical, triage, and data collection, analysis, and reporting support.[16]

In the intensivist-driven model, the critical care physician lies at the center of the team.[10] The intensivist relies on the TeleICU team members to provide key clinical information to alert them to proactively identify trends of deterioration before the impending clinical decline or patient cardiopulmonary arrest. In the TeleICU the intensivist may be responsible for the surveillance and management of upward of 100 to 250 patients.[3] At a Massachusetts academic health system, the TeleICU is staffed round the clock with intensivists who serve a primary role in managing the flow of patients into and out of the ICUs, along with providing critical care services and general supervision for APPs and residents when the managing intensivist is not available.[17] Tele-intensivist staffing ranges from 12 to 24 hours per day, depending on program design and/or need for services.[3]

The contributions and roles of APPs in the critical care workforce have been described in the literature.[18] Several organizations have integrated APP roles into their TeleICU. In these roles, Tele-APPs assess and evaluate patients using remote audio-video technologies, converse with families, provide consultation for bedside nurses, ensure adherence to best practices, and participate in care coordination and the management of unstable patients. The APP role can be invaluable in providing additional support to the tele-intensivist during high volume times in the hub.

The TeleICU nurse is usually responsible for 30 or more patients depending on the environment, level, and type of service being provided to the bedside, supporting technology, and other enabling capabilities.[3,19] The TeleICU nurse provides support to the TeleICU intensivist and to the bedside team.[2] A key function of the TeleICU nurse is to conduct ongoing reviews of large amounts of information to support the assessment and decision-making process for individual and populations of patients.[2] This function has been described as surveillance and supports the capturing, analyzing, and dissemination of relevant and clinically significant data.[19] Bedside assistance can be accomplished through support of initiatives such as assuring sedation vacations, surveying for appropriate sedation levels in ventilated patients, monitoring for the use of evidence-based best practices, or by acting as a mentor for novice ICU bedside nurses.[19] As described above, the role of the TeleICU nurse is determined by the need of the collaborative care team in caring for each site's patients.

Other clinical roles present in some TeleICUs, such as pharmacists and respiratory therapists, provide important services. For example, the pharmacist's expertise can be applied to manage vasopressors, anticoagulation medications, or deep vein thrombosis prophylaxis dosing. They may make recommendations for antibiotic de-escalation, or alert care team members to potential drug interactions as new medications are ordered. A study at a Massachusetts-based TeleICU demonstrated that pharmacists on the night shift could increase compliance with ICU sedation guidelines and extend the benefits provided by the daytime pharmacy team.[20] In Wisconsin, a TeleICU demonstrated that implementation of a remote ICU pharmacy service resulted in the provision of consistent pharmaceutical care, while minimizing costs at 13 hospitals.[21] A structured approach to glycemic control by TeleICU pharmacists at a large health system covering North and South Carolina resulted in tighter glycemic control in adult ICU patients without increasing rates of hypoglycemia.[22]

In recognizing the benefit of the pharmacist to the TeleICU team, one can begin to imagine roles for other disciplines. For example, respiratory therapists have been added to the clinical team of an independent national TeleICU provider to assist the team in the management of high-risk patients. Kacmarek[23] described that the role of the respiratory therapist in the management of mechanically ventilated patients has become paramount to providing evidence-based care of intubated patients. Kacmarek went on to describe that respiratory therapists can inform appropriate decision making related to initiation and adjustment of ventilator management, disease-specific management, analysis of ventilator waveforms, monitoring of mechanical ventilation and airway management, and assessment of diagnostic tests (laboratory and basic chest radiograph interpretation) and medication management.

GETTING TEAMS TO WORK TOGETHER: THE SYNERGY MODEL

Regardless of the specifics of team structure, some core principles must be overlaid to assure the team works effectively. The AACN TeleICU Taskforce describes how the Synergy Model for Patient Care provides a framework to enhance patient care and outcomes by matching patient characteristics/needs with nurse skill and competency.[2] AACN HWE provides criteria and standards for creating and sustaining optimal work atmospheres.[24] The Relational Coordination theoretic foundation focuses on key relationship dimensions of shared goals, shared knowledge, and mutual respect.[25] Along with the models described above, the theoretic foundation is provided that is especially relevant to TeleICU nursing practice and can be applied to all disciplines working in the TeleICU center (**Fig. 1**).[2] Clinical practice, skilled communication, collaborative relationships, and optimized technology are all characteristics that work interdependently to maintain a synergistic environment supporting the staff and the patient.[2] These interdependencies should be considered when developing workflows.[24]

COMMUNICATION IS KEY

If fee-for-service structures are to transform into a value-based oriented health care system, improved communication and true collaboration seem particularly necessary to achieve the goal of patient-focused care.[26] Communication plays a critical role in building successful teams, and patterns of communication were found to be the most important predictor of a team's success.[25] The communication between technology and the clinicians, both at the bedside and in the TeleICU, rely on the electronic medical record and various interfaces to access and track data relevant to the care of the patient. The TeleICU clinicians must use the data to forecast what may happen,

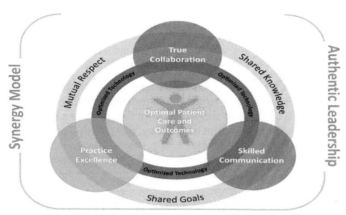

Fig. 1. AACN TeleICU nursing practice model. (*From* American Association of Critical-Care Nurses. AACN TeleICU Nursing Practice Model. AACN Tele-ICU Nursing Practice: An Expert Consensus Statement Supporting High Acuity, Progressive and Critical Care. Figure 1. Aliso Viejo (CA): American Association of Critical-Care Nurses. ©2018 by AACN. All rights reserved. Used with permission.)

design an appropriate plan in response, and then communicate those recommendations to their bedside counterparts. Communication between all the care providers must be clear and of high quality to achieve situational awareness.

Gittell described the Relational Coordination Model in which teams have shared goals, shared knowledge, and mutual respect. This leads to high-frequency communication that promotes quality collaboration resulting in patient safety and improved outcomes.[25] When there are problems or breakdowns between clinicians, the result may include preventable patient harm. The Joint Commission has found that communication issues are the most common root cause of sentinel events (serious and preventable patient harm incidents).[27]

The use of audio-visual technology as a communication tool places the remote care provider (physician, nurse, pharmacist, or APP) virtually at the bedside for visual and verbal communication and allows face-to-face dialog during the delivery of health care services.[5] A recent study by Kahn and colleagues[13] identified 3 domains as being key determinants of effective TeleICU teams in delivering improved clinical outcomes:

- Leadership: how organizational managers (ICU, TeleICU, and hospital system) make decisions about the role and reach of telemedicine.
- Perceived value: perceptions among front-line care providers about the ability of telemedicine to meaningfully improve clinical outcomes (including expectations of availability, understanding of operations, interpersonal relationships, and staff satisfaction).
- Organizational characteristics: features of the hub or distant and origin or spoke care sites that govern how remote clinical care is provided and received (such as staffing models and engagement protocols).

Kahn and colleagues[13] go on to say that programs that delivered decreases in risk-adjusted mortality after the implementation of TeleICU care tended to perform care activities in ways that were observed to be appropriate, responsive, consistent, and integrated with bedside workflows. This further validates a holistic view of the ICU team as consisting of both in-hospital and TeleICU personnel, and supports the significant emphasis on extensive communication within the team that is detailed above.

VARYING INTENSIVE CARE UNIT ENVIRONMENTS

The nature of origin care sites can differ dramatically, regardless of whether all ICUs are within a single system and especially if they are not. Key considerations that can affect the makeup of the TeleICU team include, but are not limited to

- The coverage and range of critical care expertise at the hospitals being served
- Hospital type: community or tertiary, teaching or nonteaching
- Types of ICUs to be covered and the concomitant bedside intensivist staff model
- Variations in coverage based on time of day, day of week, and/or hours of presence of intensivists at the bedside
- Whether the TeleICU is "within system" (ie, serving only hospitals within the same health system) or "trans-system" (ie, serving a range of independent and system hospitals)
- The technological capabilities that support the TeleICU
- The resources available to both the TeleICU program and each of the hospitals it serves (as scale increases, measured as number of beds, eg, additional resources or specialties, can be justified)

These factors should drive decisions related to structure, services, and team composition. The design of the TeleICU program should target the consistent delivery of high-quality care for all patients regardless of these or other variations, as measured by acuity-adjusted patient clinical outcomes, achievement of best practices, and operational considerations such as affordability and efficiency.

Most TeleICU centers begin as health system-level critical care initiatives. However, some TeleICUs serve hospitals in multiple health systems as well as individual, independent hospitals. One independent telemedicine provider, for example, was established specifically to provide TeleICU care to nonaffiliated hospitals and now supports over 75 independent and health system hospitals. In some situations, the TeleICU team augments intensivists and other critical care specialists within the hospital, whereas in others it provides the only critical care specialization.

Similarly, a large 23-hospital health system in New York has avoided a "one size fits all approach." By beginning with data collection, it imparted the technology and care model only where there was either demonstrated need based on APACHE (Acute Physiology and Chronic Health Evaluation—a standardized, risk-adjusted, severity of illness tool for ICU patients) score results or where there was expressed desire and need. Because every unit (even within the same hospital) had a different culture and staffing model, the approach to roll out and use of TeleICU was customized. This was not to say there were not standard components to be included in each new activation, but allowing key stakeholders to decide how and where this technology is implemented was essential to adaptation. In its tertiary hospitals with multiple critical care units, some units may have TeleICU coverage and others may not, depending on need and desire as described above. In other multi-ICU sites, all units may have TeleICU coverage. However, data collection surrounding outcomes is done uniformly in all units.

For some of the health system's community hospitals, the TeleICU becomes the main source of oversight starting in the late afternoon hours into the early morning. During this time there must be an APP available at the bedside capable of being the "hands" of the TeleICU intensivist. Because of the shortage of intensivists and location of some of the community hospitals, this combined staffing matrix is used differently at varying times of the day. However, what is clear is the ability of the TeleICU to support APPs at the bedside when an intensivist is not or cannot be present.

A health system located in Georgia was infused with a multimillion-dollar grant from the Centers for Medicare and Medicaid Services (CMS) in 2012 to launch a TeleICU program to support ICUs throughout Georgia.[28] This program is now providing night-time services to patients in Atlanta from Perth, Australia. This project was implemented to reduce clinician burn-out associated with working night shifts. According to a report by the CMS, the program has demonstrated reductions in the need for institutional postacute care after an ICU stay, a 2.1 percentage point decrease in 60-day readmission rates and a reduction in average spending of $1486 per 60-day episode yielding $4.6 million in Medicare savings. This health system uses APPs at the bedside supported by the TeleICU intensivists and nurses. APPs are engaged in the process of developing their role according to their scope of practice and based on the needs and perceptions of TeleICU and ICU staff.[29] APPs have the option of participating in a postgraduate residency program that has been accredited by the American Nurses Credentialing Center[30]

The aforementioned Massachusetts system has demonstrated and reported in the literature both outcome and financial benefits to using a 24/7 intensivist and APP model in its TeleICU.[17,31] Critical care nurses do not cover shifts in the TeleICU but do work collaboratively with the TeleICU providers. As mentioned previously, its Tele-ICU team serves a role in managing flow into and out of the 7 ICUs at the academic medical center. It also works with affiliated and managed care partner hospitals to provide high-level surveillance and critical care consultation services to keep patients at their home hospital when appropriate.[32]

POTENTIAL TEAM EXTENSIONS

Recently, there has been a move to include other clinical capacities in the TeleICU team. Ancillary support positions are implemented in specific TeleICUs when resources and demonstrated need exist. These positions can augment and leverage the capability of the TeleICU team and may include pharmacy, respiratory therapy, dieticians or any other position for which a need to support the bedside team can be demonstrated and financially justified. Using this core concept to leverage expertise can be highly effective in creating a systematic approach to critical care across health systems as well as across the country.

ONE OR MULTIPLE HUB SITES?

The TeleICU typically relies on centrally colocated teams, bringing all the skills into a single collaborative environment to provide care to the multiple spoke hospitals. Colocating teams in 1 place is cost-effective and creates the basis for an efficient and standardized model. However, it also introduces significant staffing risk, because all the necessary skilled TeleICU staff must be sourced in a single marketplace, which might be fraught with short supply or high competitive intensity. As an alternative, the ability to flexibly extend beyond the physical bounds of the TeleICU center and hospital can yield tremendous benefits. For example, the ability to coordinate care across multiple TeleICU centers enables recruitment of critical skills in diverse locations and can thus serve to mitigate these key risks of a single center.

In the recent merger of 2 large Midwest health systems to become a single entity, where each system has a mature TeleICU hub, a decision has been made to retain the 2 hub sites while planning to integrate and standardize the care delivery model. The benefit of this decision allows for recruitment of clinicians in both states (Illinois and Wisconsin). This widens the depth and breadth of the pool of available expertise (medical, pulmonary, surgical, trauma, neuro, anesthesia, and cardiovascular) from which to pull while establishing standard workflows in both hubs. This will assure consistency of care delivery regardless of the state from which the care is provided. The hub teams can be leveraged through cross-state licensing to establish patient assignments that may mix care between ICUs in both states to establish appropriate TeleICU workloads. In a similar example, the largest independent TeleICU care provider discussed earlier now uses a network of 9 care centers to support TeleICU care to hospitals nationwide. This enables multi-site recruiting and leverages time zone differences to mitigate local staffing risk and provide extensive system redundancy and resilience.

ADDITIONAL USES OF THE TeleICU TEAM/TECHNOLOGY

As discussed throughout, critical care is ever evolving, as are the roles and functions of the clinicians in this environment. As one considers the TeleICU team and its ability to support the interdisciplinary team, some additional methods of use could be considered as follows.

As Mentors

The use of expert TeleICU nurses to support decision making and translation of evidence-based practice has been described in the literature.[3,16,19] Experienced clinicians in the TeleICU can also be leveraged to mentor and support novice ICU clinicians. In the nursing arena, some approaches that have been taken to accomplish this include post bedside orientation mentoring and developing critical thinking skills using the TeleICU technology for novice ICU registered nurses (RNs). In one system's mentoring program, specific program objectives, structure, implementation, and evaluation are developed.[33] This allows each bedside RN who participates to feel supported in progressing from a novice nurse to an advanced beginner.

In another implementation of a critical thinking development program, new ICU RNs were given case scenarios, with the TeleICU technology integrated via screenshots to give examples of vital sign deterioration, trending in laboratories, and so forth. This allowed the novice RNs to evaluate actual patient data when making clinical care decisions. The benefit to the TeleICU in acting as the mentor is 2-fold:

1. The experienced TeleICU RN can share his or her expertise and knowledge, giving a sense of meaning to their work beyond the remote monitoring of patients; and
2. The critical relationship between caregivers on both sides of the camera, so vital to open communication and integration of the TeleICU into the ICU care team, is established and nurtured.[34,35]

TeleICU teams can offer benefits related to mentoring of residents and APPs with TeleICU intensivist oversight and remote participation in ICU sign-out.[35] During the night shift in 1 health system located in Delaware, physician assistants call the TeleICU intensivist in Illinois to discuss all new admissions and rapid response team patients. This case review provides guidance on patient management and establishes the plan of care overnight. As a side benefit to this structure for overnight partnership, these discussions and case presentations are conducted with an awake and alert TeleICU intensivist. Further, the bedside attending physician is afforded much-needed sleep, which preserves his or her sleep architecture. These models leverage the scarce resource of an attending intensivist to provide "at the end of a phone line" consultation for hundreds of patients who may be hundreds of miles away.[36] These factors, in combination, help prevent bedside physician burn-out while augmenting the development of the APPs and residents.

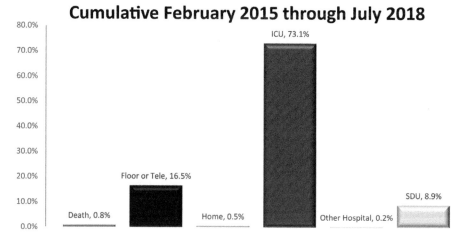

Fig. 2. eMobile cart percent by unit discharge location. (*Courtesy of* Advocate Health Care eICU.)

Real-time mentorship can extend to a variety of health care roles through experiential learning in the live TeleICU environment. Further, exposure to such programs can provide insight into the ever-changing models of patient care. Nursing students and other health care professionals in training are afforded an opportunity to glimpse their future career opportunities as experienced clinicians.

In Other Care Settings

Several TeleICU teams have extended their services in the emergency department (ED). Critical care experts in the TeleICU work with fellow team members to provide care to ICU boarders in the ED. A TeleICU in Illinois has demonstrated that, through the deployment of the TeleICU technology in the ED, about 30% of the time, patients can be admitted to a less acute level of care (floor/tele or stepdown unit) by the time a bed becomes available (**Fig. 2**). Team members working together to provide the right care at the right time results in both patient and staff satisfaction, as well as cost savings to the hospital. Other care settings for which the TeleICU technology has been leveraged include postanesthesia care units, behavioral health, disaster response, high-risk obstetrics, and to assist in timely management of patients who have had a stroke.[37]

SUMMARY

This article has discussed a framework within which to evaluate the appropriate composition and deployment of a TeleICU team in support of critically ill patients. The essential team structure combines expert clinical knowledge from both the Tele-ICU and bedside and is leveraged in a way that is flexible based on unit needs. This agility allows support that can be adapted to the individual needs of the critical care environment. Several factors must be considered when making this decision, not least of which is a method to establish consistent communication and subsequently, effective workflows to impact patient outcomes. Each organization must consider its resources (both human and financial) as well as culture and patient population needs when establishing an infrastructure.

The core principles of the AACN Synergy Model, Standards for Establishing a Healthy Work Environment and Relational Coordination provide the theoretic foundation of critical care practice. Effective communication and true collaboration play a critical role in both quality and safety when using the TeleICU model. There are opportunities to explore the effect of TeleICU mentoring and education on critical thinking capabilities of the novice nurse and other providers. There are varying TeleICU models that may be deployed depending on the goals of the organization and the components of the clinical team. Research has shown that the more integration and collaboration between the TeleICU and ICU, the greater the positive impact on patient outcomes.

TeleICU continues to be a new frontier for critical care delivery, which allows expertise to be available in a range of hospitals, enhancing quality care nationally and internationally. After nearly 2 decades of TeleICU use, there remains significant opportunity for expansion and evolution. This article has outlined how the composition and deployment of TeleICUs can be an effective and integral part of an interdisciplinary critical care team supporting the health care needs of vulnerable and complex patients where ever they are found.

REFERENCES

1. American Telemedicine Association. About Telemedicine: Q&A; 2016. Available at: http://www.americantelemed.org/main/about/telehealth-faqs-. Accessed February 27, 2017.
2. American Association of Critical Care Nurses (AACN) TeleICU Task Force. AACN TeleICU nursing practice: an expert consensus statement supporting high acuity, progressive and critical care. Aliso Viejo (CA): AACN; 2018.
3. Davis TM, Barden C, Dean S, et al. American telemedicine association guidelines for TeleICU operations. Telemed J E Health 2016;22:971–80.
4. Thomas L, Capistrant G. State telemedicine gaps analysis: coverage & reimbursement. Washington, DC: American Telemedicine Association; 2017.
5. Reynolds HN, Bander J, McCarthy M. Different systems and formats for tele-ICU coverage: designing a tele-ICU system to optimize functionality and investment. Crit Care Nurs Q 2012;35:364–77.
6. Dayal P, Hojman NM, Kissee JL, et al. Impact of telemedicine on severity of illness and outcomes among children transferred from referring emergency departments to a children's hospital PICU. Pediatr Crit Care Med 2016;17:516–21.
7. Ellenby MS, Marcin JP. The role of telemedicine in pediatric critical care. Crit Care Clin 2015;31:275–90.
8. Rogove H. How to develop a tele-ICU model? Crit Care Nurs Q 2012;35:357–63.
9. Goran SF. A new view: tele-intensive care unit competencies. Crit Care Nurse 2011;31:17–29.
10. Lilly CM, Zubrow MT, Kempner KM, et al. Critical care telemedicine: evolution and state of the art. Crit Care Med 2014;42:2429–36.
11. Rosenfeld BA, Dorman T, Breslow MJ, et al. Intensive care unit telemedicine: alternate paradigm for providing continuous intensivist care. Crit Care Med 2000;28:3925–31.
12. Kim MM, Barnato AE, Angus DC, et al. The effect of multidisciplinary care teams on intensive care unit mortality. Arch Intern Med 2010;170:369–76.
13. Kahn JM, Rak KJ, Kuza CC, et al. Determinants of intensive care unit telemedicine effectiveness: an ethnographic study. Am J Respir Crit Care Med 2018. https://doi.org/10.1164/rccm.201802-0259OC.

14. Udeh C, Udeh B, Rahman N, et al. Telemedicine/virtual ICU: where are we and where are we going? Methodist Debakey Cardiovasc J 2018;14:126–33.

15. Kahn JM, Le TQ, Barnato AE, et al. ICU telemedicine and critical care mortality: a national effectiveness study. Med Care 2016;54:319–25.

16. Goran SF. A second set of eyes: an introduction to Tele-ICU. Crit Care Nurse 2010;30:46–55.

17. Lilly CM, Motzkus C, Rincon T, et al. ICU telemedicine program financial outcomes. Chest 2017;151:286–97.

18. Buchman T, Boyle W, Beyatte M. Shaping the next critical care workforce. In: Kleinpell RM, Boyle WA, Buchman TG, editors. Integrating nurse practitioners & physician assistants into the ICU: strategies for optimizing contributions to care. Mount Prospect (IL): Society of Critical Care Medicine; 2012.

19. Rincon TA, Henneman E. An introduction to nursing surveillance in the tele-ICU. Nurs Crit Care 2018;13:42–6.

20. Forni A, Skehan N, Hartman CA, et al. Evaluation of the impact of a tele-ICU pharmacist on the management of sedation in critically ill mechanically ventilated patients. Ann Pharmacother 2010;44:432–8.

21. Meidl TM, Woller TW, Iglar AM, et al. Implementation of pharmacy services in a telemedicine intensive care unit. Am J Health Syst Pharm 2008;65:1464–9.

22. Everhart S, Kosmisky D, Karvetski C, et al. Tele-ICU Pharmacist Impact on Glycemic Control Across a Large Healthcare System. 2016 ASHP Best Practice Award; 2016. Available at: https://www.ashp.org/About-ASHP. Accessed November 12, 2018.

23. Kacmarek RM. Mechanical ventilation competencies of the respiratory therapist in 2015 and beyond. Respir Care 2013;58:1087–96.

24. American Association of Critical Care Nurses (AACN). AACN standards for establishing and maintaining healthy work environments. Aliso Viejo (CA): AACN; 2016.

25. Gittell JH, Godfrey M, Thistlethwaite J. Interprofessional collaborative practice and relational coordination: improving healthcare through relationships. J Interprof Care 2013;27:210–3.

26. McCauley K, Irwin RS. Changing the work environment in intensive care units to achieve patient-focused care: the time has come. Am J Crit Care 2006;15:541–8.

27. Patient Safety Network (PSNet). Communication Between Clinicians. Patient Safety Primer; 2018. Available at: https://psnet.ahrq.gov/primers/primer/26/Communication-Between-Clinicians. Accessed November 12, 2018.

28. Woodruff Health Sciences Center. Emory cares for ICU patients remotely, turning 'night into day' from Australia. Emory News Center; 2018. Available at: https://news.emory.edu/stories/2018/05/buchman-hiddleson_eicu_perth_australia/index.html. Accessed November 12, 2018.

29. Leventhal R. Emory healthcare saves $4.6M with tele-ICU program. Healthcare Informatics; 2017. Available at: https://www.healthcare-informatics.com/news-item/telemedicine/emory-healthcare-saves-46m-tele-icu-program. Accessed November 12, 2018.

30. American Nurses Credentialing Center (ANCC). Emory critical care center nurse practitioner residency program: gaining accreditation to better support nurse practitioners. Silver Spring (MD): ANCC; 2015.

31. Lilly C, Cody S, Zhao H, et al. Hospital mortality, length of stay, and preventable complications among critically ill patients before and after tele-ICU reengineering of critical care processes. JAMA 2011;305:E1–9.

32. New England Healthcare Institute and Massachusetts Technology Collaborative. Tele-ICUs: remote management in intensive care units. Cambridge (MA): New England Healthcare Institute (NEHI); 2007. p. 1–37.

33. Brindise T, Baker MP, Juarez P. Development of a tele-ICU postorientation support program for bedside nurses. Crit Care Nurse 2015;35:e8–16.

34. Mullen-Fortino M, DiMartino J, Entrikin L, et al. Bedside nurses' perceptions of intensive care unit telemedicine. Am J Crit Care 2012;21:24–31 [quiz: 2].

35. Venditti A, Ronk C, Kopenhaver T, et al. Tele-ICU "Myth Busters". AACN Adv Crit Care 2012;23:302–11.

36. Goran SF, Mullen-Fortino M. Partnership for a healthy work environment: tele-ICU/ICU collaborative. AACN Adv Crit Care 2012;23:289–301.

37. Healthcare P. eICU program: Telehealth for the intensive care unit. Philips Enterprise telehealth; 2017. Available at: https://www.usa.philips.com/healthcare/product/HCNOCTN503/eicu-program-telehealth-for-the-intensive-care-unit. Accessed October 21, 2017.

UNITED STATES POSTAL SERVICE®

Statement of Ownership, Management, and Circulation
(All Periodicals Publications Except Requester Publications)

1. Publication Title	2. Publication Number	3. Filing Date
CRITICAL CARE NURSING CLINICS OF NORTH AMERICA	006 – 273	9/18/21

4. Issue Frequency	5. Number of Issues Published Annually	6. Annual Subscription Price
MAR, JUN, SEP, DEC	4	$160.00

7. Complete Mailing Address of Known Office of Publication (Not printer) (Street, city, county, state, and ZIP+4®)

ELSEVIER INC.
230 Park Avenue, Suite 800
New York, NY 10169

Contact Person: Malathi Samayan
Telephone (Include area code): 91-44-4299-4507

8. Complete Mailing Address of Headquarters or General Business Office of Publisher (Not printer)

ELSEVIER INC.
230 Park Avenue, Suite 800
New York, NY 10169

9. Full Names and Complete Mailing Addresses of Publisher, Editor, and Managing Editor (Do not leave blank)

Publisher (Name and complete mailing address)
DOLORES MELONI, ELSEVIER INC.
1600 JOHN F KENNEDY BLVD. SUITE 1800
PHILADELPHIA, PA 19103-2899

Editor (Name and complete mailing address)
KERRY HOLLAND, ELSEVIER INC.
1600 JOHN F KENNEDY BLVD. SUITE 1800
PHILADELPHIA, PA 19103-2899

Managing Editor (Name and complete mailing address)
PATRICK MANLEY, ELSEVIER INC.
1600 JOHN F KENNEDY BLVD. SUITE 1800
PHILADELPHIA, PA 19103-2899

10. Owner (Do not leave blank. If the publication is owned by a corporation, give the name and address of the corporation immediately followed by the names and addresses of all stockholders owning or holding 1 percent or more of the total amount of stock. If not owned by a corporation, give the names and addresses of the individual owners. If owned by a partnership or other unincorporated firm, give its name and address as well as those of each individual owner. If the publication is published by a nonprofit organization, give its name and address.)

Full Name	Complete Mailing Address
WHOLLY OWNED SUBSIDIARY OF REED/ELSEVIER, US HOLDINGS	1600 JOHN F KENNEDY BLVD. SUITE 1800 PHILADELPHIA, PA 19103-2899

11. Known Bondholders, Mortgagees, and Other Security Holders Owning or Holding 1 Percent or More of Total Amount of Bonds, Mortgages, or Other Securities. If none, check box ▶ ☐ None

Full Name	Complete Mailing Address
N/A	

12. Tax Status (For completion by nonprofit organizations authorized to mail at nonprofit rates) (Check one)
The purpose, function, and nonprofit status of this organization and the exempt status for federal income tax purposes:
☒ Has Not Changed During Preceding 12 Months
☐ Has Changed During Preceding 12 Months (Publisher must submit explanation of change with this statement)

PS Form **3526**, July 2014 [Page 1 of 4 (see instructions page 4)] PSN: 7530-01-000-9931   PRIVACY NOTICE: See our privacy policy on www.usps.com.

---

13. Publication Title	14. Issue Date for Circulation Data Below
CRITICAL CARE NURSING CLINICS OF NORTH AMERICA	JUNE 2021

15. Extent and Nature of Circulation			Average No. Copies Each Issue During Preceding 12 Months	No. Copies of Single Issue Published Nearest to Filing Date
a. Total Number of Copies (Net press run)			137	112
b. Paid Circulation (By Mail and Outside the Mail)	(1)	Mailed Outside-County Paid Subscriptions Stated on PS Form 3541 (Include paid distribution above nominal rate, advertiser's proof copies, and exchange copies)	78	57
	(2)	Mailed In-County Paid Subscriptions Stated on PS Form 3541 (Include paid distribution above nominal rate, advertiser's proof copies, and exchange copies)	0	0
	(3)	Paid Distribution Outside the Mails Including Sales Through Dealers and Carriers, Street Vendors, Counter Sales, and Other Paid Distribution Outside USPS®	26	25
	(4)	Paid Distribution by Other Classes of Mail Through the USPS (e.g., First-Class Mail®)	0	0
c. Total Paid Distribution (Sum of 15b (1), (2), (3), and (4))			104	82
d. Free or Nominal Rate Distribution (By Mail and Outside the Mail)	(1)	Free or Nominal Rate Outside-County Copies included on PS Form 3541	18	16
	(2)	Free or Nominal Rate In-County Copies included on PS Form 3541	0	0
	(3)	Free or Nominal Rate Copies Mailed at Other Classes Through the USPS (e.g., First-Class Mail)	0	0
	(4)	Free or Nominal Rate Distribution Outside the Mail (Carriers or other means)	0	0
e. Total Free or Nominal Rate Distribution (Sum of 15d (1), (2), (3) and (4))			18	16
f. Total Distribution (Sum of 15c and 15e)			122	98
g. Copies not Distributed (See Instructions to Publishers #4 (page 43))			15	14
h. Total (Sum of 15f and g)			137	112
i. Percent Paid (15c divided by 15f times 100)			85.24%	83.67%

* If you are claiming electronic copies, go to line 16 on page 3. If you are not claiming electronic copies, skip to line 17 on page 3.

16. Electronic Copy Circulation	Average No. Copies Each Issue During Preceding 12 Months	No. Copies of Single Issue Published Nearest to Filing Date
a. Paid Electronic Copies		
b. Total Paid Print Copies (Line 15c) + Paid Electronic Copies (Line 16a)		
c. Total Print Distribution (Line 15f) + Paid Electronic Copies (Line 16a)		
d. Percent Paid (Both Print & Electronic Copies) (16b divided by 16c × 100)		

☒ I certify that 50% of all my distributed copies (electronic and print) are paid above a nominal price.

17. Publication of Statement of Ownership
☒ If the publication is a general publication, publication of this statement is required. Will be printed in the DECEMBER 2021 issue of this publication. ☐ Publication not required.

18. Signature and Title of Editor, Publisher, Business Manager, or Owner

Malathi Samayan - Distribution Controller   *Malathi Samayan*   Date 9/18/21

I certify that all information furnished on this form is true and complete. I understand that anyone who furnishes false or misleading information on this form or who omits material or information requested on the form may be subject to criminal sanctions (including fines and imprisonment) and/or civil sanctions (including civil penalties).

PS Form **3526**, July 2014 (Page 2 of 4)   PRIVACY NOTICE: See our privacy policy on www.usps.com

Moving?

Make sure your subscription moves with you!

To notify us of your new address, find your **Clinics Account Number** (located on your mailing label above your name), and contact customer service at:

Email: journalscustomerservice-usa@elsevier.com

800-654-2452 (subscribers in the U.S. & Canada)
314-447-8871 (subscribers outside of the U.S. & Canada)

Fax number: 314-447-8029

Elsevier Health Sciences Division
Subscription Customer Service
3251 Riverport Lane
Maryland Heights, MO 63043

Printed and bound by CPI Group (UK) Ltd, Croydon, CR0 4YY

03/10/2024

01040408-0009